# THE POWER OF LOVE
# A NURSING THEORY

### WHEN SCIENCE MEETS SPIRIT. A NEW KIND OF NURSE IS BORN

**WINSTON MEIKLE**

MSN, MBA, RN

Copyright © 2025 by WINSTON MEIKLE

All Rights Reserved

LCCN: 2025938615

# Table of Contents

Introduction ................................................................. 1

    Love + Mind = Holistic Healing ................................. 4

    Core Principles of the New Nursing Theory: ............. 7

    A Practice Rooted in the Loving, Intelligent, Energetic Universe ................................................................. 7

Chapter 1: The Evolution of Nursing Theories ................ 12

    About Nursing ....................................................... 12

    Nursing Theories ................................................... 12

    Nursing Theorists .................................................. 13

    Why Are Nursing Theories Important? ................... 14

    Purposes of Nursing Theories ............................... 16

    Classification of Nursing Theories ......................... 16

    Significant Milestones in The Evolution of Nursing ..... 18

    Early Nursing Theories .......................................... 18

    Mid-20th Century ................................................... 19

    Humanistic and Holistic Approaches ..................... 20

    Systems and Adaptation Theories ......................... 20

    Contemporary Theories ......................................... 21

Current Trends and Future Directions.......................... 21

Chapter 2: The Power of Positive & Intentional Thinking 28

    Awareness ................................................................ 30

    Nursing & Love – Brief Overview ............................... 32

    Positive Thinking ........................................................ 33

    Watson's 10 Carative Factors .................................... 35

    Assumptions .............................................................. 35

    Strengths ................................................................... 35

    Weakness .................................................................. 36

    The Science Behind Positive Thinking ....................... 37

        Cultivating a Positive Mindset ................................ 38

        Navigating Negative Thought Patterns ................... 38

        Building Positive Relationships .............................. 38

        The Long-Term Impact of Positive Thinking ............ 39

        The Benefits of Positive Thinking ............................ 39

    5 Scientific Studies that Prove the Power of Positive Thinking ................................................................................ 40

        1.   Study on the Power of Positive Visualizations .. 40

        2.   Study Showing Happiness Leads to Success ... 41

        3.   Study on Stress and the Immune System ......... 41

        4.   Penn Resilience Program ................................. 41

5. The Nun Study on Longevity ............................ 42
Positive Thinking and the Brain ................................ 42
The Science of Affirmations ...................................... 43
    The Brain's Response to Positive Thinking ............. 43
    What Is the Science Behind Positive Affirmations? . 44
    The Science Behind Affirmations: How Effective Are They? ............................................................................ 45
The Neuroscience Behind Positive Thinking .............. 45
Positive Thinking and Physical Health ....................... 47
Positive Thinking and Mental Health .......................... 47

Chapter 3: Quantum Physics and the Inter-connected Web of Healing Energy! ....................................................... 49
    Quantum Physics ...................................................... 50
    Quantum Mechanics ................................................. 51
    Principles of Quantum Physics ................................. 51
        1. Superposition: ................................................. 52
        2. Entanglement: ................................................. 52
        3. Observation: ................................................... 52
    An Experiment That Raises More Questions Than It Answers ..................................................................... 52
        Quantum Entanglement ........................................ 52

Applying These Concepts to Nursing Care Delivery 55

The Non-Locality of the Physical Reality .................... 56

Dr. Masaru Emoto's Work in the Context of Quantum Physics and Entanglement............................................. 57

The Power of Thought and Healing ........................... 58

Applying Quantum Physics Principles in Nursing Practice ................................................................... 58

    1. Holistic Care: .................................................. 59

    2. Energy Healing: .............................................. 59

    3. Mind-Body Connection: ................................... 59

    4. Patient-Centered Care: .................................... 59

    5. Telehealth: ...................................................... 59

    6. Preventative Care: ........................................... 59

    7. Interdisciplinary Collaboration: .......................... 60

Quantum Physics and Healing.................................. 62

The Paradigm Shift in Healthcare ............................. 63

Quantum Physics and Nursing Research .................. 63

The Unified Field Theory and What Heals ................. 64

Integrating Quantum Principles into Clinical Practice . 69

Quantum Reality, Universal Love, and Nursing Theory .................................................................................. 70

Future Implications for Nursing Theory ...... 72

References ............... 75

Chapter 4: The Power of Intention and Visualization ...... 77

Overview ............ 77

What is Intention? ............ 80

McTaggart, L - The Intention Experiment ............ 80

Dr. Masaru Emoto's Water Studies ............ 81

In the Context of Nursing: ............ 83

What is Visualization & Imagery? ............ 85

How to? ............ 85

Visualization in Healthcare & Nursing ............ 86

The Relationship Between the Mind, Body and Consciousness ............ 89

Intention, Visualization, and the New Thought Authors ............ 90

The Power of Manifestation ............ 92

The Law of Assumption ............ 93

The Power of Imagination ............ 95

How to Manifest in Five Steps ............ 95

Jean Watson's Carative Principles and the Power of Intention & Visualization ............ 97

References .................................................................. 101

Chapter 5: THE BUTTERFLY EFFECT ........................ 103

    Overview.................................................................. 103

    What is the Butterfly Effect?..................................... 105

        The Butterfly Flap in the Healing Space ................ 106

        Scientific Bridges: Chaos, Energy, and Entanglement ................................................................................ 107

        Where the Butterfly Danced – Some Micro and Macro Instances ................................................................. 108

    The Butterfly Effect of Caring .................................. 109

        1.   Patient Interactions and Outcomes: ................ 110

        2.   Systemic Changes and Health Outcomes: ...... 110

        3.   Emotional and Psychological Effects: .............. 110

        4.   Holistic Care and the Ripple Effect: .................. 111

    Conclusion .............................................................. 112

Chapter 6: Case Studies in Mind-Body Healing ........... 115

    Wim Hof's Method ................................................... 115

        Cold Exposure: ..................................................... 116

        Breathing: ............................................................. 117

        Meditation: ............................................................ 117

    Health Benefits of the Wim Hof's Method ............... 118

Implications for Nursing Practice .............................. 119

    Case Study 1: Chronic Pain Management ............ 119

    Case Study 2: Anxiety Management ...................... 120

Wim Hof Method Teaching Plan: ............................... 120

Joe Dispenza's Work on Mind-Body Connection and Its Implications on Nursing ................................................ 122

    The Core of Dr. Joe Dispenza's Philosophy .......... 123

    Mind-body connection: ........................................... 123

    Meditation and mindfulness: ................................... 124

    Self-Awareness and Personal Transformation: ..... 124

    How Dr. Joe Dispenza's Approach Can Facilitate Healing ............................................................................ 125

    References ............................................................... 127

Chapter 7: Emotions and Health .................................. 128

    Human Emotions and the Human Body .................... 129

    How Emotions Affect Your Physical Health ............... 130

    The Connection between Positive Psychology and Nursing: ............................................................................ 133

    Positive Relationships lead to Healthier Living. ......... 134

    Emotions in Nursing Practice & Healthcare ............... 134

    Emotions, Prayer, and Healing: ................................. 135

The Emotion of Love and Healing: ............................ 138

Conclusion ................................................................ 140

References .............................................................. 141

Chapter 8: The Role of Nutrition in Healthcare & Nursing
............................................................................... 143

   Diet and Lifestyle ..................................................... 144

   The Role of Micronutrients ...................................... 148

   Impact of Nutrition on Chronic Diseases .................. 148

      Importance of a Balanced Diet ............................ 148

   Biohacking and Optimal Health ............................... 149

      Biohacking ............................................................ 149

      Optimal Health ..................................................... 149

      Brendon Burchard ............................................... 150

      Ben Greenfield ..................................................... 151

      Tim Ferriss ........................................................... 151

   FDA's Role in the Safety of the American Food Supply
............................................................................... 152

   The Role of Nutrition in Healthcare .......................... 156

   Nutrition and Its Role in Nursing Practice ................ 159

      Principles of Nutrition in Nursing Practice ............. 159

      Importance of Nutrition in Nursing Practice ........... 160

The Role of Nutrition in Disease Prevention ............. 162

Nutrition and the Mind-Gut Connection ..................... 163

    Nutrition & Cognition: ........................................... 164

    The Role of a Nurse in Promoting Proper Health .. 165

Practicing Self-Care ................................................. 168

Strategies for Improving Nutrition in Clinical Settings 169

Devil's Advocate ...................................................... 170

Conclusion ............................................................... 171

References ............................................................... 172

Chapter 9: Mindfulness and Nursing Practice .............. 174

    What is Mindfulness? ............................................... 176

    Mindfulness and Orem's Self-Care Deficit Theory .... 177

        Core Concepts of the Self-Care Deficit Theory: .... 178

        Application in Nursing Practice .............................. 179

    Mind-Body Connection and Healing ......................... 180

    Modulation of Anxiety by Expectations ..................... 184

    Holistic Approach to Patient Care ............................ 184

    Joe Dispenza and Gregg Braden on the Superpower: PLAECBO ................................................................ 185

    The Nocebo Effect ................................................... 188

    Mindful Self-care for Nurses .................................... 189

Conclusion .................................................................. 192

References ................................................................ 194

**Chapter 10: HEALING ACROSS CULTURES** ............... 196

1. Traditional Chinese Medicine (TCM) and Other Healing Traditions ........................................................... 197

    The Chi Gung Master of Malaysia ........................ 197

    Relevance to Nursing and Patient Care ............... 198

2. Hinduism - Prana ................................................ 199

    Spanda .................................................................. 200

3. Hawaiian Culture – Mana – The Life Force of Healing 201

4. Native American Culture - Spirit ......................... 207

Shamanism and Its Relevance to Nursing Practice .. 207

    Relevance to Nursing Practice ............................. 208

Challenges and Ethical Considerations .................... 209

    Evidence-Based Applications ............................... 209

Chi Kung Master DJ Healer and His Approach to Healing through Positive Thought ............................................. 209

    Application to Nursing and Patient Care: ............. 211

    Some More Healing Practices Across Cultures ........ 212

Importance of Cultural Sensitivity in Healthcare and Healing .................................................................... 213

    Conclusion ............................................................ 215

    References ........................................................... 217

  Conclusion ................................................................ 219

# Introduction

The idea that *"our thoughts create our reality while our emotions attract it"* resonates with principles found in various philosophical, psychological, and spiritual frameworks. Our thoughts influence how we interpret and respond to the world. If we think positively about a challenge, we are more likely to take proactive steps, creating outcomes aligned with that mindset. Psychologically, our thoughts shape our beliefs, which drive our actions and behaviors, influencing the outcomes we experience. This aligns with the concepts of "mental rehearsal" and visualization, where envisioning success leads to subconscious alignment with that goal. *Contemporary scientific and philosophical perspectives suggest that reality is fundamentally energetic, with all Matter existing in various vibrational states. Within this framework, thoughts can be conceptualized as subtle energetic forms that interact with broader energetic fields, including what is described in quantum physics as the quantum field. However, the relationship between cognition, perception, and physical reality is complex and extends beyond oversimplified interpretations.*

*The human unconscious mind plays a crucial role in shaping human perception and behavior. Empirical research in cognitive science and psychology indicates that subconscious processes govern a significant proportion of human decision-making and interactions with the external world. Some estimates suggest that up to 95% of cognitive activity occurs beyond conscious awareness, influencing beliefs, behaviors, and perceptions of reality. This highlights the profound role of subconscious conditioning in structuring an individual's experience of the world.*

*Expanding upon the connection between thought and the quantum field, it is essential to recognize the dynamic interplay between different energetic states. The quantum field, as understood in modern physics, describes a fundamental level of reality where particles and waves exist in superpositions and probabilities until influenced by observation or interaction. While the extent to which consciousness directly affects the quantum field remains a topic of debate, studies in fields such as quantum cognition and mind-matter interaction propose mechanisms through which mental states might correlate with physical outcomes. In this context, thoughts may be viewed as energetic influences that resonate within a broader field of interactions, potentially influencing both subjective experience and material reality.*

*Further interdisciplinary research is required to bridge insights from physics, neuroscience, and consciousness studies to refine our understanding of these interactions.* Quantum Physics and the Unified Field Theory affirm this mysterious phenomenon of how everything is interconnected and holds the power to influence and transform the other. *Quantum physics principles suggest that our thoughts influence not only our emotional states and biological processes within the body but also extend their impact to the objectively observable physical reality beyond the body.*

As per the Law of Attraction, emotionally charged thoughts—those we feel deeply—are believed to have a magnetic quality that attracts similar vibrations or circumstances. For example, a state of gratitude can often draw more reasons to feel grateful. Emotions influence our body language, tone, and actions, influencing how others interact with us and the opportunities we encounter. Our brain seeks consistency between our emotional state and the external world. For instance, a positive mood can lead to more positive interactions, perpetuating a cycle. Do you see the relevance to healing and human care here?

We also know that emotions are the energy behind our intentions. They amplify the signals we send into the world, influencing how people perceive and respond to us. When you feel joy or gratitude, you radiate positivity, which attracts similar experiences and interactions. Conversely, unresolved negative emotions can lead to self-sabotage or strained relationships. So, we can assume that thoughts and emotions do not act in isolation. Thoughts and emotions allow us to navigate, adapt, and transform our experiences. A healed human being is a product of a healthy collaboration between inner mastery, i.e., cultivating positive, aligned thoughts and emotions, and outer action, i.e., taking practical steps in the external world.

Some cultures and traditions worldwide align closely with the belief that our thoughts and emotions influence reality. However, it extends the concept into a spiritual and interconnected worldview. Shamanism, for instance, emphasizes the interconnectedness of all things—mind, body, spirit, and the external world—making it deeply resonant with ideas about co-creating reality through intention and energy.

Emotions, in such traditions, are perceived as energetic frequencies that align us with certain outcomes or spirits. For example, emotions like gratitude or reverence are seen as harmonizing energies that attract guidance, healing, or abundance from the realm of *collective consciousness*. Practices like drumming, chanting, and dancing heighten emotional states and connect with desired energies. Shamans work with the energy of individuals and their environment. This reflects the idea that emotions (energy in motion) can influence the vibrational patterns around us, shaping the reality we experience. Shamanism teaches that humans are deeply connected to nature, spirits, and universal energy. This perspective supports the belief that thoughts and emotions ripple through this interconnected web, affecting personal reality and the collective experience.

Practices like mindfulness, meditation, and visualization allow the mind to regulate stress responses, reduce pain, and promote overall well-being. A growth-oriented mindset and mental practices like gratitude or reframing negative experiences could miraculously help individuals recover from emotional challenges and setbacks. Loving-kindness meditation or embracing unconditional love is tied to enhanced mental clarity, reduced anxiety, and greater emotional balance. The mind is a central tool in both directing and facilitating healing through focus, belief, and intention. The brain's ability to rewire itself means that positive thoughts and mental practices can create new, healthier neural pathways, fostering emotional and physical healing. The power of belief, a function of the mind, can trigger fundamental physiological changes. This demonstrates how our thoughts and expectations influence our body's healing processes.

### Love + Mind = Holistic Healing

When love and the mind work together, their healing potential is amplified. For example, compassion-focused therapy combines emotional warmth (love) with mental reprogramming for trauma recovery. At the same time, loving mindfulness practices could integrate self-compassion and cognitive awareness, promoting deep healing for the soul, body, and mind. Applying the healing powers of **Love and the Mind** to nursing practice could transform patient care, enhance resilience among nurses, and foster a compassionate healthcare environment.

The profession of nursing has undergone significant changes and advancements over the years. Nursing theories and practices have continuously evolved from the days of Florence Nightingale to modern-day nursing practices. However, there has been little focus on the power of the mind and the force of love in nursing practice. This book aims to bridge this gap by introducing a new nursing theory based on the power of the mind and the force of love, supported by quantum physics and the unified field theory.

The nursing theory presented in this book integrates elements from prominent nursing theorists such as Florence Nightingale, Martha Rogers, Jean Watson, Dorothea Orem, Madeline Leininger, Pender, Henderson, Imogene King, and Kalista Roy. It combines these theories with insights from mindful thinking, quantum physics, and influential works by new thought authors. The theory is further supported by Dr. Masaru Emoto's water studies, the practices of Wim Hoff and Steven Kotler, and the teachings of Napoleon Hill and Joe Dispenza. Additionally, the book draws on examples across cultures, including Chi Kung Master DJ healer, shamanism, and the placebo effect.

This book systematically incorporates mindful thinking, empathy, and compassion into nursing practice to enhance patient outcomes and create meaningful life experiences. It emphasizes the role of positive thinking in fostering healing and improving the work environment for nurses. Practical examples and tools are provided to integrate mindfulness into nursing care, highlighting the significance of love and compassion in the healing process.

The book also explores mind-body healing practices from different cultures, such as Chi Gung, shamanism, and the practices of the Hunza people of the Himalayas. It is structured into over a dozen chapters, covering a wide range of topics, including the evolution of nursing theories, the mind-body connection, mindfulness and meditation techniques, the power of intention and visualization, the influence of emotions on health outcomes, the placebo effect, case studies in mind-body healing, the role of nutrition and exercise, creating a healing environment, self-care for nurses, incorporating positive thinking into nursing education, and the future of nursing and the power of love.

The evidence supporting the power of positive thinking and mindfulness across scientific disciplines is substantial, as is the proof of the healing effects of love. From the placebo effect to the works of new thought, authors like Napoleon Hill and Rhonda Byrne, a prominent figure in research, support the idea that our thoughts and beliefs significantly impact our physical and mental well-being.

This book proposes an advanced theory of Nursing based on Love and the power of the Human Mind to heal, supported by scientific research, spiritual traditions, and anecdotal evidence. The New Nursing Theory advocates that Love and the Human Mind are potent forces influencing our physical, emotional, and psychological well-being, often profoundly and in a transformative way.

Love—whether self-love, interpersonal love, or universal love—has been shown to foster healing in several ways. Love nurtures feelings of safety, connection, and acceptance, essential for overcoming trauma, reducing stress, and promoting emotional resilience. This theory highlights the importance of consciousness, positive thought, the mystery of the Life Force and its manifestations and healing abilities, and its interplay with physical reality and how that works within the Nursing practice.

The New Nursing Theory emphasizes the power of 'self-talk' and how negative self-talk in patients could be fatal in extreme cases. However, the focus is not merely on the power of self-talk but on the fundamental energetic reality in which we exist and how our thoughts react with this interconnected field. Self-talk serves as one mechanism for directing intentions and attuning to the unified or universal field of love. Mind over matter underscores the ability to shape reality through thoughts, intentions, emotions, words, and actions that align with this energetic framework, facilitating manifestation and transformation. Correspondingly, in Nursing practice or healthcare, a positive self-talk narrative could carry healing properties and fast-track a patient's recovery. These are known and observed phenomena that can now be wielded by conscious approaches to the idea of mind over matter and manifesting our reality through thoughts and words. Practices like Reiki have scratched the surface of this phenomenon of the dynamic interplay of energies and consciousness as applied to energetic interventions to create beneficial outcomes.

This book is a comprehensive and practical guide for integrating the power of the mind and love into nursing practices. By adopting a systematic approach to mindful thinking, nurses can enhance patient outcomes, improve their well-being, and contribute to advancing the nursing profession by all means.

## Core Principles of the New Nursing Theory:

### A Practice Rooted in the Loving, Intelligent, Energetic Universe

In the sacred unfolding of modern nursing, a new paradigm emerges—one that sees the nurse not merely as a caregiver but as a conduit of healing energy, a steward of consciousness, and a partner in co-creation. This theory rests upon nine foundational principles, each serving as an invitation to deepen, expand, and elevate nursing practice into a sacred art.

#### 1. The Principle of Energetic Unity

At the heart of existence lies a simple truth: all is energy. Every person, every thought, every cell pulses with vibration, woven into a vast, intelligent matrix of being. The nurse and the patient are not separate; they are participants in a shared field of resonance. When a nurse enters the room with a calm heart and a centered mind, healing begins—often before a word is spoken. This principle calls nurses to become conscious of their energetic presence, cultivating practices that align best with body, mind, and spirit. Through touch, tone, presence, and intention, they transmit more than care—they transmit coherence. In honoring the sacred interconnectedness of all life, nurses' midwives harmonize with the spaces they inhabit.

## 2. The Principle of Conscious Intent

Every intention is a seed. When planted in awareness, it grows into outcomes that ripple through energy fields, altering the course of healing. The principle of conscious intent teaches that the nurse's inner world is not separate from the clinical environment—it shapes it. Whether through a silent prayer before entering a room or a quiet affirmation whispered in the heart, intention becomes a subtle yet powerful medicine. When nurses guide patients to set their own healing intentions, the therapeutic encounter transforms into a co-creative partnership. Healing ceases to be something done to the patient, and becomes a journey with them, authored by both will and wonder.

## 3. The Principle of Loving Intelligence

Beneath the surface of all creation flows a current of loving intelligence—a divine consciousness that expresses itself through care, compassion, and the quiet wisdom of the heart. In this model, nursing transcends protocol and becomes poetry. The nurse, attuned to the whispers of intuition, becomes a vessel through which this sacred intelligence speaks. Sometimes it guides the hand. Sometimes it holds the silence. It always honors the patient's soul, seeing not just the illness, but the wholeness that lies beneath. Through this lens, every act of care is a dialogue between the sacred and the seen, the infinite and the embodied.

### 4. The Principle of Resonance and Vibration

Healing is harmony restored. Each individual emits a frequency, and when that frequency is coherent, resonant with love, peace, and vitality, health naturally follows. The nurse, through cultivated self-awareness, becomes a tuning fork of healing. A soothing voice, a peaceful presence, a gentle gaze—these are not incidental. They are frequencies transmitted. Nurses who are attuned to high-vibration states uplift the entire care environment. They surround patients with sound, color, scent, and sacred space, creating environments where the body remembers how to heal. In this principle, nursing is not only clinical—it is musical. It is vibrational medicine.

### 5. The Principle of Perception as Reality

What we believe, we become. Perception is vital in shaping the biology, influencing the very cells that construct our lived reality. A nurse guided by this principle becomes a weaver of narrative, gently reframing the patient's inner story from fear to empowerment. Through language, presence, and trust, the nurse helps patients see themselves not as broken, but as becoming. Education is no longer just instruction—it is illumination. When a patient perceives their own strength, healing accelerates. The nurse becomes both mirror and lighthouse, reflecting potential and lighting the path ahead.

### 6. The Principle of Self as Healer

Within every person lives an innate healer—a quiet force of regeneration and rebalance. The nurse's role is not to fix, but to awaken this intelligence. By witnessing the patient as already whole, the nurse activates dormant potential. Self-care practices—breath, stillness, nourishment, movement—are not supplementary; they are essential rituals of reclamation. As nurses model these practices in their lives, they embody the message: you are your medicine. In this sacred partnership, the nurse is not the hero, but the guide, holding space while the patient rediscovers the healing wisdom within.

## 7. The Principle of Co-Creation

Healing is never a solo act. It is the symphony of many hands, hearts, and intentions coming together in a dance of possibility. The nurse honors the patient's voice, the family's wisdom, the team's skills, and the environment's soul. All are contributors. All are creators. In this dynamic field of cooperation, outcomes are shaped not by hierarchy but by harmony. The nurse facilitates this sacred gathering, encouraging shared decisions, collective rituals, and a unified vision. Healing, then, is not only personal—it is communal.

## 8. The Principle of Present-Moment Awareness

The now is holy. It is where breath lives, where intuition speaks, where healing unfolds. Nurses anchored in the present moment become portals of peace, helping patients ground in the here and now, where pain can be eased, fear quieted, and life felt more fully. Mindful breathing, compassionate presence, and deep listening are not luxuries in care; they are its essence. As the nurse dwells fully in each moment, they draw patients into that sacred presence, where suffering softens and grace arrives. The present moment becomes a temple of transformation.

## 9. The Principle of Sacred Service

Nursing is not merely a profession; it's a call from within. It is sacred work, rooted in reverence for life and devotion to love. When a nurse approaches each task—whether complex or mundane—with humility, compassion, and awareness, it becomes a prayer in motion. Sacred service does not burn out; it burns bright. It is sustained by purpose, grounded in self-care, and guided by something greater. In this light, the nurse becomes a bridge between worlds—where science meets spirit, and care becomes ceremony.

In embracing these nine principles, the nurse steps into a new archetype: not just as a healer but as a harmonizer, co-creator, and sacred presence. The future of nursing, then, is not only more compassionate but more conscious. And in that consciousness, the true art of healing is reborn.

# Chapter 1: The Evolution of Nursing Theories

*A Brief Overview*

## About Nursing

Nursing, as a profession, is dedicated to recognizing its own peculiar body of knowledge crucial to nursing practice or nursing science. To distinguish this foundation of knowledge, nurses need to identify, develop, and understand concepts and theories related to nursing. Nursing is a science based on the theory of what it actually is, what nurses do, and why. It is a unique discipline separate from medicine, with its own distinct body of knowledge and a focus on holistic care that is different from the disease-centered approach of medicine.

Nursing has undergone a profound transformation since the days of Florence Nightingale. It has evolved from a basic, simple care profession to a complex, multi-faceted field focusing on providing holistic care. This evolution has been mirrored in the development of nursing theories, each building on the work of its predecessors.

## Nursing Theories

Nursing theories are not just abstract concepts; they are organized bodies of knowledge that define what nursing is, what nurses do, and why they do it. They serve as a practical framework, guiding nursing practice at a more concrete and specific level and distinguishing nursing as a unique discipline separate from other fields, such as medicine. These theories are not just theoretical constructs but are applied in real-life nursing situations, guiding nurses in their daily interactions with patients and in their approach to patient care.

Nursing theories are the basis of nursing practice today. In many cases, nursing theory guides knowledge development and directs education, research, and practice. Historically, nursing was not recognized as an academic discipline or a profession as we view it today. Before nursing theories were developed, nursing was considered a task-oriented occupation. The training and function of nurses were under the direction and control of the medical profession.

The evolution of nursing theories has not only shaped the nursing field but also significantly influenced workplace cultures, perspectives, methodologies, and emphases over time. These theories provide a framework for nursing practice, guiding nurses in their interactions with patients, their understanding of healthcare environments, and their approach to patient care. Each new theory builds on the work of its predecessors, further shaping the field and the cultures within it.

## Nursing Theorists

Most Nurse Theorists did not create a Nursing Theory[i] but constructed a way to improve caregiving and the relationship between the caregiver and the care recipient. Most theorists had to give up their personal lives to stay true to the profession and invest with all their might. They had well-rounded educational backgrounds and varied interests. Their inquisitive nature and self-reliance made them stand out in making a difference both in the field and in the lives of their clients.

# Why Are Nursing Theories Important?

Nursing theories are integral to nursing, providing a structured framework that guides practice, research, and education. Here's a detailed exploration of their significance:

1. **Foundation of Practice**: Nursing theories establish the foundation for nursing practice by clearly defining what nursing is and what it should entail. They help nurses understand their roles, responsibilities, and the unique contributions they make to the healthcare system.

2. **Guiding Nursing Interventions**: Theories offer a scientific rationale for nursing interventions, equipping nurses with a knowledge base that informs their actions and decisions in various clinical situations. This ensures that care is delivered in a consistent and evidence-based manner.

3. **Shaping Future Directions**: Nursing theories provide a conceptual framework, contributing to developing nursing knowledge and indicating how the profession should evolve. This continuous advancement is crucial for addressing emerging challenges in healthcare.

4. **Professional Identity and Recognition**: Nursing theories give nurses a sense of identity within the healthcare environment. They help other healthcare professionals, patients, and administrators recognize and appreciate nurses' distinct roles in patient care.

5. **Critical Reflection and Knowledge Expansion**: Theories encourage nurses to reflect on their practice critically, question existing assumptions, and explore the underlying values of their profession. This reflective practice not only

deepens the understanding of nursing but also expands its knowledge base.

6. **Research and Evidence-Based Practice**: Nursing theories guide research and inform evidence-based practice. They provide a framework for generating research questions, testing hypotheses, and interpreting findings, ultimately improving patient care and outcomes.

7. **Communication and Common Language**: Nursing theories facilitate effective communication among nurses and other healthcare professionals by providing a common language and set of concepts. This shared understanding is essential for collaboration and the delivery of coordinated care.

8. **Educational Development**: Nursing theories are a basis for developing nursing education and training programs. They inform curriculum design, teaching methodologies, and assessment criteria, ensuring that nursing students are well-prepared to meet the profession's demands.

9. **Defining and Predicting Nursing Phenomena**: Theories aim to define, predict, and explain nursing phenomena, helping to standardize care practices and improve the quality of care. They also help maintain nursing professional boundaries, ensuring the discipline remains distinct and respected within the broader healthcare landscape.

10. **Continuous Professional Growth**: Nursing theories help bridge the gap between academic knowledge and clinical practice by linking theory, practice, and research in a continuous, reciprocal relationship. This ongoing interaction promotes theory-guided practice, enhancing the profession's ability to meet societal needs.

## Purposes of Nursing Theories

The primary goal of nursing theory is to enhance practice by improving patient health outcomes and quality of life. These theories are essential for advancing nursing as an academic discipline, a field of research, and a profession. They help define and describe nursing care, guide practice, and provide a foundation for clinical decision-making.

- **In Academic Discipline**: Nursing theories have historically shaped nursing education, providing a structured framework for building curricula. This helps articulate the profession's core values and principles, enhancing its academic and professional status.

- **In Research**: Theories are fundamental to the research process, providing a framework that guides the study of nursing phenomena. This interplay between theory, research, and practice is vital for closing the gap between theoretical knowledge and practical application.

- **In the Profession**: In clinical settings, nursing theories encourage reflection, questioning, and critical thinking, helping nurses to understand and improve their practice. This reflective practice is essential in a field where tradition and institutional forces often dominate.

## Classification of Nursing Theories

Nursing theories can be classified based on their level of abstraction, goal orientation, or underlying philosophical assumptions:

- **By Abstraction**:

- **Grand Nursing Theories**: Broad and abstract, these theories provide a general framework but do not guide specific interventions.

- **Middle-Range Nursing Theories**: More focused and testable, these theories address specific phenomena and are often derived from grand theories.

- **Practice-Level Nursing Theories**: Narrow in scope, these theories are situation-specific and directly inform nursing interventions and outcomes.

- **By Goal Orientation**:
  - **Descriptive Theories**: These theories describe and explain nursing phenomena without necessarily guiding actions.
  - **Prescriptive Theories**: These theories are action-oriented, guiding nursing interventions and predicting outcomes.

- **By Philosophical Underpinnings**:
  - **Needs-Based Theories**: Focus on fulfilling patients' physical and mental needs.
  - **Interaction Theories**: Emphasize the nurse-patient relationship and the impact of the environment.
  - **Outcome Theories**: Focus on the control and direction of patient care based on physiological and behavioral knowledge.

Nursing theories are vital to the development of the nursing profession. They provide great insights, structure, and tools to advance practice, research, and education. They are essential for maintaining the profession's professional integrity and ensuring that it continues to evolve in response to society's changing needs.

# Significant Milestones in The Evolution of Nursing

## Early Nursing Theories

Nursing theory is the backbone of the nursing profession. It provides a framework for nurses to understand and approach patient care. Nursing theory is an organized set of concepts, definitions, and assumptions that explain or describe the phenomenon of nursing. It helps nurses identify and define what they do, why they do it, and the expected outcomes of their actions. Nursing theory development is a continuous process that has evolved, influenced by different perspectives and experiences.

The first nursing theories appeared in the late 1800s when nursing education was strongly emphasized. Theory development and Research were an integral part of modern nursing.

**Florence Nightingale (1859)**

**Environmental Theory:** Often considered the founder of modern nursing, Florence Nightingale's work during the Crimean War highlighted the importance of a clean environment, fresh air, and proper sanitation in patient recovery. Her theory emphasized the nurse's role in manipulating the environment to aid healing. In 1860, Florence Nightingale defined nursing in her "Environmental Theory" as "utilizing the patient's environment to assist him in his recovery."

# Mid-20th Century

In the 1950s, nursing scholars agreed that nursing needed to validate itself by producing scientifically tested knowledge.

### Hildegard Peplau (1952)

**Interpersonal Relations Theory:** Peplau introduced the concept of the nurse-patient relationship, focusing on the therapeutic interaction between the nurse and the patient. Her theory emphasized communication and the importance of understanding patient behavior to provide effective care. In 1952, Hildegard Peplau introduced her Theory of Interpersonal Relations, emphasizing the nurse-client relationship as the foundation of nursing practice.

In the 1960s, the first doctoral programs in nursing were established (Chinn & Kramer, 1999) due to the realization that Nursing was unique and contained aspects that other disciplines, such as Sociology, Psychology, etc., did not. Nursing was found to be distinctive as it revolved around managing humans in various states of wellness i.e., the mental, social, spiritual, and psychosocial aspects.

### Virginia Henderson (1966)

**Need Theory:** Henderson identified 14 basic needs of individuals that nursing care should address, ranging from physiological needs to self-actualization. Her theory underscored the nurse's role in assisting patients with activities contributing to health, recovery, or a peaceful death.

**In 1968, Dorothy Johnson pioneered the Behavioral System Model** and upheld the fostering of efficient and effective behavioral functioning in patients to prevent illness.

In 1971, Imogene King's Theory of Goal attainment stated that the nurse is considered part of the patient's environment and the nurse-patient relationship is for meeting goals towards good health.

## Humanistic and Holistic Approaches

### Madeleine Leininger (1978)

**Transcultural Nursing Theory:** Leininger highlighted the importance of cultural competence in nursing care. Her theory stressed the need for nurses to understand and respect the cultural backgrounds of patients to provide culturally congruent care.

### Jean Watson (1979)

**Theory of Human Caring:** Watson's theory emphasized the humanistic aspects of nursing combined with scientific knowledge. She introduced the concept of "carative factors" as a guide for the core of nursing, focusing on the importance of caring relationships and patients' subjective experiences. **In 1979,** Jean Watson developed the philosophy of caring and highlighted humanistic aspects of nursing as they intertwine with scientific knowledge and nursing practice.

## Systems and Adaptation Theories

### Dorothea Orem (1971)

**Self-Care Deficit Theory:** Orem's theory focuses on the individual's ability to perform self-care and the nurse's role in supporting patients to meet their self-care needs. She identified self-care requisites and the importance of teaching patients to manage their health independently.

**Sister Callista Roy (1970)**

**Adaptation Model:** Roy's model views patients as adaptive systems that cope well with environmental changes. The nurse's role is to help patients adapt to these changes, promoting their overall health and well-being.

## Contemporary Theories

**Patricia Benner (1984)**

**From Novice to Expert:** Benner's theory describes the stages of clinical competence that nurses go through, from novice to expert. Her work emphasized the importance of experiential learning and the development of clinical skills over time.

**Nola Pender (1982)**

**Health Promotion Model:** Pender's model focuses on the proactive pursuit of health and well-being. Her theory emphasized the role of nurses in promoting healthy behaviors and lifestyle changes to prevent illness and enhance patients' quality of life.

## Current Trends and Future Directions

Over the past century, nursing theory has undergone significant evolution. Early nursing theories were rooted in the medical model, focusing on specific nursing actions to improve patient outcomes. However, as nursing established itself as a distinct discipline, theorists began to explore what makes nursing unique from medicine.

In recent years, nursing theory has also expanded to explore the influence of the mind and the power of love in promoting health and healing. This emerging perspective is supported by evidence from studies on positive thinking and mindfulness across various scientific disciplines. It draws on concepts from quantum physics, such as the double-slit experiment and unified field theory. The work of new thought authors like Dr. Masaru Emoto, who studied the effects of consciousness on water, and contributions from Wim Hof, Steven Kotler, Napoleon Hill, Joe Dispenza, and Rhonda Byrne have all enriched this evolving area of nursing theory.

Nursing theory became integral to the discipline as nursing became a recognized profession. It provides a framework for understanding and organizing nursing knowledge, which helps nurses make informed decisions, guides nursing practice, and supports research. Nursing theories are also crucial for educating future nurses and developing curricula that reflect the profession's core principles.

Nursing theory has been vital in developing nursing as a profession. It has provided a foundation for practice, education, and research, helping nurses better understand the unique aspects of their work. Nursing theory will likely be crucial in shaping the discipline's future as nursing evolves.

**Integrative and Evidence-Based Practice**

The contemporary focus in nursing theory is on integrating various theoretical perspectives and applying evidence-based practices. This approach combines the best aspects of different theories to provide comprehensive, patient-centered care.

**Technology and Informatics**

Integrating technology and informatics into nursing practice is an increasingly important area of focus. Theories in this field examine how technological advancements can enhance patient care, improve health outcomes, and support the nursing profession.

**Unitary Caring Science**

It represents an elevated level of thought that extends beyond traditional Caring Science. It is grounded in the 'Ethic of Belonging,' inspired by Levinas' philosophy, and prioritizes this ethic before the individualistic Ontology of Being. The concept of Belonging within the boundless realm of universal cosmic Love serves as the ethical foundation for our understanding of Being. Our human experiences, as we navigate the sacred cycle of life and death, are intertwined within this infinite, universal field of Cosmic Love (Levinas, 1969; Watson, 2005, 2008, 2018).

Unitary Caring Science encourages an expanded and evolving worldview that embraces the idea of Unitary or ALL, aligning with Rogers' Science of Unitary Human Beings. Research within Unitary Caring Science explores reflective, subjective, and interpretive inquiries alongside objective-empirical approaches, including sacred action as a form of inquiry. It welcomes and integrates ontological, philosophical, ethical, spiritual, and historical inquiries and other emerging fields of study.

**The Healing Power of Love in Nursing: A Foundation in Watson's Caring Science[ii]**

Watson's Caring Science is an evolving philosophical-ethical field rooted in nursing, which extends beyond conventional Western science to embrace a holistic, relational approach to healing. First introduced in *Nursing: The Philosophy and Science of Caring* (1979), this theory emphasizes the integration of mind, body, and spirit, viewing the person as a unified whole connected with their environment.

Central to Caring Science is the recognition of metaphysical phenomena such as love, spirit, and consciousness, which are vital to the healing process. This theory advocates for a unitary perspective, where love is seen as a universal, cosmic force that transcends time and space, connecting individuals at a deeper, spiritual level.

In nursing, the practice of love manifests through the *10 Caritas Processes®*, which guide nurses in creating caring relationships that foster healing beyond the physical. These processes include sustaining humanistic values through loving-kindness, developing trusting relationships, and being authentically present with patients. Through these practices, nurses engage in transpersonal caring, which not only addresses the immediate needs of patients but also nurtures their inner life and spiritual well-being.

This approach calls for a shift from a purely technological focus on curing disease to a more comprehensive model that integrates the art of caring and the science of healing. By centering their consciousness and intentionality on love and caring, nurses can create healing environments that honor the whole person, facilitating not just physical recovery but also emotional and spiritual growth.

In this framework, love is not just an emotion but a vital force that empowers nurses to connect deeply with their patients, offering them comfort, hope, and a sense of belonging. This transcendent love is the cornerstone of healing, making nursing a profound and transformative practice that touches the soul as much as it heals the body.

**Glossary**

Nursing theory development demands an understanding of selected terminologies, definitions, and assumptions.

**Philosophy.** These are the beliefs and values that define a way of thinking and are generally known and understood by a group or discipline.

**Theory.** A belief, policy, or procedure proposed or followed as the basis of action. It refers to a logical group of general propositions used as principles of explanation. Theories are also used to describe, predict, or control phenomena.

**Concept.** Concepts are often called the building blocks of theories. They are primarily the vehicles of thought that involve images.

**Models.** Models are representations of the interaction among and between the concepts, showing patterns. They present an overview of the theory's thinking and may demonstrate how the theory can be introduced into practice.

**Conceptual framework.** A conceptual framework is a group of related ideas, statements, or concepts. It is often used interchangeably with the **conceptual model** and with **grand theories**.

**Proposition.** Propositions are statements that describe the relationship between the concepts.

**Domain.** The domain is the perspective or territory of a profession or discipline.

**Process.** Processes are organized steps, changes, or functions to achieve the desired result.

**Paradigm.** A paradigm refers to a pattern of shared understanding and assumptions about reality and the world, worldview, or widely accepted value system.

**Metaparadigm.** A metaparadigm is the most general statement of a discipline and functions as a framework in which the more restricted structures of conceptual models develop. Much of the theoretical work in nursing focused on articulating relationships among four major concepts: person, environment, health, and nursing.

**References:**

Alligood, M. R. (2014). Nursing theorists and their work. Elsevier Health Sciences.

McEwen, M., & Wills, E. M. (2014). Theoretical basis for nursing. Lippincott Williams & Wilkins.

Newman, M. A. (2014). Health as expanding consciousness. Jones & Bartlett Publishers.

Rogers, M. E. (1992). Nursing: Science of unitary, irreducible human beings: In three parts. Appleton & Lange.

Watson, J. (2008). Nursing: The philosophy and science of caring (revised edition). University Press of Colorado.

For Chapter 1: The Historical Evolution of Nursing Science:

Feeley, A. M. (2017). A perspective on the development of nursing science: past, present, and future. Nursing Science Quarterly, 30(4), 306-310. https://doi.org/10.1177/0894318417720209

Fawcett, J., Watson, J., Neuman, B., Walker, P. H., & Fitzpatrick, J. J. (2015). On nursing theories and evidence. Journal of Nursing Scholarship, 47(6), 545-547. https://doi.org/10.1111/jnu.12173

Parse, R. R. (2016). Nursing science and the space-time continuum. Nursing Science Quarterly, 29(1), 6–7. https://doi.org/10.1177/0894318415623002

Brown, C. G. (2017). Nursing science: The foundation for evidence-based practice. Nursing Science Quarterly, 30(2), 94–97. https://doi.org/10.1177/0894318417699267

# Chapter 2: The Power of Positive & Intentional Thinking

*Thoughts are matter in motion and have the energy to wield our reality. Thoughts can be understood as dynamic forms of energy capable of influencing reality.* Thoughts are not supernal or celestial. They are representations of matter and are encoded in matter. They have shape and weight. Abstract ideas are analogically built from more concrete sensory representations or maps. [iii]The concepts of Transmission of Thought and State Transference or the Hive Brain are not new. What we think, we create; what we feel, we make a reality. Energy flows, where focus goes. When like-minded individuals come together with a shared intention, they create a potent collective energy field. This energy catalyzes positive change within the group and the world at large. *Within an intelligent and conscious universe, thoughts manifest as tangible entities. At the subatomic level, physicality becomes less dominant, while consciousness assumes a more significant role, as evidenced by principles in quantum physics and the unified field theory."*

Our thoughts are like the architects of our inner world. They shape our perspectives, intentions, and actions. When we focus on empowering thoughts, we align our behaviors with those ideas, increasing the likelihood of achieving desired outcomes. For example, believing in your ability to succeed can fuel the effort and resilience needed to make it happen. Fundamentally, our thoughts are maps representing and corresponding to things that our brains have either perceived with our senses, felt with our emotions, or formed as an action plan (e.g., creating an image of reaching for ripe fruit on a tree branch). All of these are electrochemically mediated processes. Thoughts indeed hold the power to guide us toward either a successful path or one of self-destruction.

To create positive momentum in our lives, we must practice intentional thinking[iv]. This involves being mindful of our thoughts and having the courage to challenge them. By effectively challenging our thoughts and differentiating them from emotions, we can take control of our lives and steer them in a positive direction. For instance, there are times when we might 'Feel' unworthy, thereby 'Thinking' that we truly ARE unworthy. Let us challenge that thought. Even though we feel unworthy, there is a concept called *'intentional thinking'*, which helps us recognize that this *'Feeling'* does NOT define our worth. It is just an emotion, rooted in childhood, originating from someone else's insecurity and having nothing to do with who we indeed are. Our intentional thinking helps us realize that the feeling is not valid and is connected to our old baggage.

The brain is an energy-intensive organ, consuming 20% of the body's energy at rest despite only accounting for 2% of the body's weight. The brain's energy consumption increases during cognitively demanding tasks. When the energies align, interactions occur. The more precise the alignment, the more responsive the energies are to each other. [v] Energy and mass are interchangeable ($E=mc^2$), meaning that the energy transmitting a thought has mass. The ions and molecules encoding this energetic signal have mass, too. While it might be possible to calculate the weight of a single thought, the number would be infinitesimally small but not zero.

The power of Imagination is a force to be reckoned with. Harnessing its power to get and live the desired life, our thoughts and feelings shape our reality based on our chosen psychological states. Believing in the power of our imagination to manifest physical outcomes, impressing our unconscious mind with thoughts and feelings, leads to the manifestation of desired outcomes, and various other teachings affirm and validate the Healing and Manifesting power of the Mind and the Feeling of Love.[vi]

Our body heals faster when conscious thought and underlying beliefs support the process. We cannot deny that our thoughts consistently or constantly flow into our states and actions. To enable healing, one must start by letting go of what does not serve or help the healing process. Doubts, mistrust, or feelings of despair and grief could hamper the process of healing in any person, and it has to happen in both the caregiver and the care recipient.

The power of belief in already having what is desired for manifestation and the difficulty transitioning between different states of consciousness and their effect on interactions are other ways to expedite healing in patients and people in every walk of life. The transition from pursuing business growth to consulting due to changing desires, acquiring clients who stay true to their desires and achieve significant success, and then emphasizing the importance of following personal desires over external appearances are all helpful ideas.

## Awareness

Awareness is vital to manifesting any thought or transfer in any state. Prayer, for instance, is an art that requires practice to manifest desirable experiences and learn from different states. *A higher concentration of aligned thoughts and collective prayers can significantly influence physical reality. This phenomenon is supported by various studies, including the random number generator experiment, which affirms a correlation between collective human intention and measurable physical outcomes.*

Collective thoughts and intentions can influence physical reality, which was proved by the RNG[1] Experiment, or the Global Consciousness Project, led by Dr. Roger Nelson at Princeton University. It studied whether collective human intention could

---

[1] Random Number Generator

influence random number generators (RNGs). RNGS produce sequences of numbers that should be entirely random under normal conditions. During globally significant events (e.g., 9/11 attacks, New Year's Eve, Princess Diana's funeral), deviations in the randomness of the RNGS were recorded. These deviations were statistically significant, suggesting a correlation between collective emotional focus and changes in physical systems. The said study was conclusive that the collective consciousness of humanity might create a measurable influence on physical systems.

These experiments and studies suggest a profound connection between collective human intention and physical reality. Whether through influencing randomness, societal conditions, or biological systems, these phenomena highlight the potential power of focused thought and collective consciousness to shape the physical world.

The conscious mind reasons inductively from observation, experience, and education to reveal subconscious assumptions; hence, bringing awareness to our thoughts and feelings allows us to release identification and manifest from a desired premise. By recognizing and letting go of negative thoughts to create space for positive manifestations, one can align one's thoughts with one's desired outcomes. Beliefs play an integral role in manifestation. Believing one already has what one desires is crucial for manifesting one's reality.

Practicing mindfulness and self-awareness effectively transitions between different states of consciousness. This can ease the transition and align with desired outcomes. It is important to follow personal desires over external appearances because personal desires align with our true selves and lead to authentic fulfillment and success. Prayer helps manifest desirable experiences because it influences the unconscious mind to accept desired outcomes, paving the way for their manifestation.

The significance of bringing awareness to our thoughts and feelings is that awareness allows us to release limiting beliefs and manifest them from a desired premise. Practice transmutation techniques to affirm and manifest your desires in reality. Our minds act like a mirror. It reflects our thoughts through our experiences and interactions with others. Their unconscious mind picks up what we think and feel about someone, even if they are not physically present.

As Tesla said, we are beings of energy and habit. If we wish to understand the universe, we must think about it in terms of energy, frequencies, and vibrations. Humans and beings of nature transmit vibes and perceive and exchange energies to communicate. We are energetic beings in an energetic universe, and thoughts are just one way energy is expressed. Aligning energies by actively choosing and precisely choosing the matching emotional, energetic state with the right thought and emotion activates the manifestation of physical response.

## Nursing & Love – Brief Overview

In Nursing, the New Nursing Theory posits that Love is a fundamental force that connects all living beings in the universe. It believes that the energy of love promotes healing, growth, and transformation in individuals, communities, and the environment. Love is a fundamental force that unites all entities within the universe, both living and non-living. The entire cosmos exists as a conscious, intelligent, and energetic field where various forms of energy interact to shape what we perceive as reality. The Law of Attraction can be understood as a manifestation of this energetic framework, reflecting the intelligent consciousness embedded within the unified field that underlies all existence. Individuals can harmonize with this field through intentional alignment, positive thinking, and love.

Love, the unified field, and the concept of God can be regarded as interchangeable, as consciousness is the foundation of all existence, and love represents its most profound and powerful expression. The theory affirms that nursing should focus on nurturing and promoting love in patients, families, and communities. The law of attraction affirms that positive thoughts and emotions attract positive experiences, while negative thoughts and emotions attract negative experiences. Nursing theory integrates these concepts and confirms that promoting love and positive energy in patients can influence their gene expression, brain function, and overall health and well-being.

The New Nursing theory also emphasizes the importance of a holistic approach to nursing care, considering the patient care's physical, emotional, spiritual, and social aspects. It encourages nurses to be mindful of their energy and promotes self-care to cultivate positive energy and love in themselves and their patients.

## Positive Thinking[vii]

The new nursing theory speculates that love is a potent force for healing and transformation, asserting that fostering love and positive energy in patients is fundamental to nursing practice. This concept aligns with the ideas presented in "The Power," a self-help book by Rhonda Byrne, published in 2010,[viii] which explores the "law of attraction." The book contends that positive thoughts and emotions attract favorable experiences, whereas negative thoughts and emotions attract unfavorable ones. Byrne argues that individuals can harness the power of positive thinking to realize their desires and achieve their goals, suggesting that a shift in one's thoughts and emotions can lead to significant life changes. The book provides practical techniques and exercises aimed at helping readers cultivate positive energy to attract success and happiness.

The nursing theory discussed here integrates the law of attraction concept, proposing that nurses can positively influence patients' health and well-being by promoting positive energy and love. The theory further emphasizes the significance of self-care and mindfulness in nurturing positive energy. However, expert analysis highlights that the law of attraction lacks scientific validation and may be subject to limitations. While positive thinking and emotions can enhance overall well-being, they do not guarantee success or happiness in every situation. Experts also caution against overly simplistic interpretations of the law of attraction, which may overlook critical external factors such as socioeconomic status, structural inequalities, and systemic barriers that impact individuals' lives.

Nonetheless, the proposed nursing theory acknowledges the intricacy of nursing care, advocating for a holistic approach that considers the physical, emotional, spiritual, and social dimensions of health and well-being. By fostering love and positive energy in patients and prioritizing self-care and mindfulness, nurses can contribute to positive thinking or maintaining an optimistic outlook, which involves consciously focusing on the positive aspects of any situation. This mindset can significantly influence both physical and mental health. However, it's important to note that positive thinking doesn't mean ignoring reality or downplaying challenges. Instead, it's about approaching life's ups and downs with the expectation that things can improve.

The impact of positive thinking has been widely acknowledged and extensively studied, with research exploring its effects on various facets of life. This mindset is marked by an emphasis on finding the good in every situation, grounded in the belief that optimistic thoughts can lead to better outcomes. In nursing, positive thinking can be a powerful asset, helping to enhance patient care and boost patient outcomes. This chapter will explore the scientific evidence from various disciplines that support the effectiveness of positive thinking in healthcare.

## Watson's 10 Carative Factors

These are: (1) forming humanistic-altruistic value systems, (2) instilling faith-hope, (3) cultivating a sensitivity to self and others, (4) developing a helping-trust relationship, (5) promoting an expression of feelings, (6) using problem-solving for decision-making, (7) promoting teaching-learning, (8) promoting a supportive environment, (9) assisting with the gratification of human needs, and (10) allowing for existential-phenomenological forces. The first three factors form the "philosophical foundation" for the science of caring, and the remaining seven come from that foundation.

## Assumptions

Watson's model makes seven assumptions: (1) Caring can be effectively demonstrated and practiced only interpersonally. (2) Caring consists of carative factors that result in the satisfaction of specific human needs. (3) Effective caring promotes health and individual or family growth. (4) Caring responses accept the patient as he or she is now and what he or she may become. (5) A caring environment offers potential development while allowing patients to choose the best action for themselves at a given time. (6) The science of caring is complementary to the science of curing. (7) The practice of caring is central to nursing.

## Strengths

Although some consider Watson's theory complex, many find it easy to understand. The model can guide and improve practice, equipping healthcare providers with the most satisfying aspects of practice and providing the client with holistic care. Watson considered using nontechnical, sophisticated, fluid, and evolutionary language to artfully describe her concepts, such as caring love, carative factors, and Caritas. Paradoxically, abstract and simple concepts such as caring love are difficult to practice, yet practicing and experiencing them leads to greater understanding.

Also, the theory is logical because the carative factors are based on broad assumptions that provide a supportive framework. The carative factors are logically derived from the assumptions and related to the hierarchy of needs. Watson's theory is best understood as a moral and philosophical basis for nursing. The scope of the framework encompasses broad aspects of health-illness phenomena. Also, the theory addresses aspects of health promotion, preventing illness, and experiencing peaceful death, thereby increasing its generality. The carative factors provide guidelines for nurse-patient interactions, an important aspect of patient care.

## Weakness

The theory does not furnish explicit direction about how to achieve authentic caring-healing relationships. Nurses who want concrete guidelines may not feel secure using this theory alone. Some have suggested that it takes too much time to incorporate the Caritas into practice, and some note that Watson's emphasis on personal growth is a quality "that while appealing to some may not appeal to others."

Watson's theory provides a valuable and essential metaphysical orientation for the delivery of nursing care. Watson's theoretical concepts, such as the use of self, patient-identified needs, the caring process, and the spiritual sense of being human, may help nurses and their patients find meaning and harmony during a time of increasing complexity. Watson's rich and varied knowledge of philosophy, the arts, the human sciences, and traditional science and traditions, along with her prolific ability to communicate, has enabled professionals in many disciplines to share and recognize her work.[ix]

## The Science Behind Positive Thinking[x]

In an era filled with unpredictability and challenges, maintaining a positive mindset is not just beneficial; it is essential for navigating the complexities of modern life. This exploration into the art of positive thinking focuses on its importance during tough times, emphasizing how a shift in perspective can impact mental, emotional, and physical well-being, leading to personal and professional growth.

**Neurological Benefits**: Positive thinking is not just a feel-good mantra; it is rooted in science. Optimism can rewire brain pathways, reducing the production of stress hormones and boosting mood-enhancing chemicals like serotonin and dopamine. This neurological shift enhances mental well-being and contributes to better physical health.

**Physical Health Advantages**: A positive mindset is linked to improved health outcomes. It can lower the risk of chronic diseases, aid in faster recovery, and potentially increase lifespan. Optimism boosts the immune system, making the body more resilient against illnesses.

**Psychological Resilience**: Positive thinking is a key component in developing psychological resilience. This resilience allows individuals to rebound from setbacks more effectively, viewing challenges as opportunities for growth rather than insurmountable obstacles.

## Cultivating a Positive Mindset

Mindfulness and Meditation Techniques are trends and tools for fostering a centered, positive mindset. They help cultivate present-moment awareness, reduce stress, and enhance overall well-being. Expressing gratitude, whether through journaling or verbal acknowledgment, shifts focus from what is lacking to what is abundant in our lives, fostering a more positive outlook. Regular practice of positive affirmations and visualization can reinforce a hopeful outlook and manifest positive changes. They are powerful tools in shaping one's mindset and outlook on life.

## Navigating Negative Thought Patterns

Learning to recognize and reframe negative thoughts is crucial in cultivating a positive mindset. It is about changing the narrative from a pessimistic viewpoint to an optimistic one. Cognitive-behavioral techniques effectively alter entrenched negative thought processes. They involve identifying distorted thinking and gradually reshaping it toward more positive, realistic thoughts. Professional counseling or therapy is sometimes necessary to manage persistent negative thinking. It provides a structured approach to understanding and altering deep-rooted negative thought patterns.

## Building Positive Relationships

It is essential to surround oneself with people who encourage and support positive thinking. These relationships can significantly impact one's outlook on life. Managing and minimizing the impact of negative influences is crucial for maintaining a positive mindset. This might involve setting boundaries or limiting interactions with those who drain emotional energy.

## The Long-Term Impact of Positive Thinking

A consistent positive outlook can lead to long-term happiness, fulfillment, and achievement. The benefits of positive thinking aren't just transient; they can shape one's life. Various studies and research findings support the long-term benefits of a positive mindset. These scientific validations offer a compelling reason to embrace positive thinking as a way of life.

## The Benefits of Positive Thinking

Many studies have looked at the role of optimism and positive thinking in mental and physical health. It's not always clear what comes first: the mindset of these benefits. But there is no downside to staying upbeat.

Some physical benefits may include:

- Longer life span
- Lower chance of having a heart attack
- Better physical health
- Greater resistance to illnesses such as the common cold
- Lower blood pressure
- Better stress management
- Better pain tolerance

The mental benefits may include:

- More creativity
- Greater problem-solving skill
- Clearer thinking
- Better mood
- Better coping skills
- Less depression

When individuals in one study were exposed to the flu and common cold, those who maintained a positive outlook were less likely to fall ill and reported experiencing fewer symptoms. In another study, women with a more optimistic mindset had a lower risk of death from cancer, heart disease, stroke, respiratory disease, and infection. Additionally, research involving people over 50 found that those with more positive beliefs about aging tended to live longer. They also exhibited reduced stress-related inflammation, suggesting a potential link between their mindset and overall health. It's worth noting that people with a positive outlook may be more inclined to adopt healthy lifestyle habits due to their hopeful perspective on the future. However, even after researchers accounted for this factor, the positive correlation between optimism and health outcomes remained significant.

# 5 Scientific Studies that Prove the Power of Positive Thinking[xi]

Happier people tend to live longer, enjoy better health, and achieve greater success in life. Instead of seeking external sources of happiness, adopting a scientific approach to cultivating happiness can be more effective. By learning to replace negative, hopeless thoughts with positive imagery or feelings, we can significantly boost our chances of happiness. While this might sound like pop psychology, it is supported by scientific evidence. Here are five studies published in peer-reviewed journals that demonstrate the power of positive thinking:

### 1. Study on the Power of Positive Visualizations

In a study published in the *Journal of Behavior Research and Therapy* in March 2016, researchers from King's College London tested 102 individuals diagnosed with anxiety disorder. Participants were divided into three groups: one group visualized a positive outcome for three specific worries from the past week, another group thought of verbal positive outcomes, and the final group visualized any positive image whenever they started to worry. The two groups that practiced positive visualization, whether related to specific worries or not, reported increased happiness, better rest, and reduced anxiety.

## 2. Study Showing Happiness Leads to Success

A review published in the December 2005 issue of *Psychological Bulletin* examined studies involving over 275,000 people and found that the happiest individuals partly owe their success to their optimism and positive outlook. Dr. Lyubomirsky, the lead researcher from UC Riverside, concluded, "When people feel happy, they tend to be confident, optimistic, and energetic, and others find them likable and sociable." These traits help happy people capitalize on positive perceptions, contributing to success.

## 3. Study on Stress and the Immune System

Researchers led by Dr. Segerstrom at the University of Kentucky analyzed over 300 studies conducted in the past 30 years on the effects of stress. They found that short-term stress provides a burst of adrenaline, strengthening the immune system and helping individuals manage immediate challenges. However, chronic stress weakens the immune system over time, leading to illness, depression, and anxiety disorders. The takeaway: changing your thinking about it is essential if you can't change a stressful situation.

## 4. Penn Resilience Program

Based on decades of research, the Penn Resilience Program has been shown to help schoolchildren, college students, and even soldiers in the U.S. Army build resilience against stress and anxiety. The program teaches coping mechanisms and strategies to enhance positivity in emotional, social, spiritual, and family well-being, helping participants better manage stress or trauma. The U.S. Army now uses this program as a preventive measure against PTSD.

### 5. The Nun Study on Longevity

Researchers from the University of Kentucky conducted a study examining autobiographies written in the 1930s by nuns who lived together in the same convent during their early years between the ages of 18 and 32. These writings were rated for positivity. Sixty years later, the researchers followed up with the surviving nuns, aged 75 to 90. They found that the nuns who had lived beyond the average life expectancy scored high on positive thoughts or feelings in their early writings, regardless of their circumstances.

These studies collectively highlight the profound impact that positive thinking can have on mental health, resilience, and overall well-being.

## Positive Thinking and the Brain

*The idea that we live in an **energetic, intelligent, and conscious universe** aligns with various scientific, philosophical, and spiritual understandings. Quantum physics affirms that at the most fundamental level, everything is energy vibrating at different frequencies. Consciousness is a fundamental aspect of reality rather than just a byproduct of the brain.*

*The interaction of energies and their vibrations shapes the physical and ethereal realms since thoughts, emotions, and intentions carry energetic frequencies that influence reality. This also ties into the **law of resonance**—that we attract and interact with energies similar to our own vibrational state.*

Numerous studies have demonstrated that positive thinking can influence the brain's structure and function, which has significant implications for healing and nursing care. Positive thoughts are linked to proficiency and enhanced productivity in the prefrontal cortex, a region responsible for essential cognitive functions such as decision-making and problem-solving. Additionally, positive thinking has been associated with heightened activity in the brain's reward centers, including the amygdala and striatum, which play key roles in pleasure and motivation.

In one study, individuals trained to think positively showed increased gray matter volume in the right inferior parietal cortex, an area involved in self-awareness and self-reflection. Another study revealed that those who practiced loving-kindness meditation, which emphasizes positive feelings toward oneself and others, experienced increased activity in the left prefrontal cortex. This region is associated with positive emotions and self-referential processing.

These findings underscore the potential of positive thinking as a therapeutic tool in nursing, where fostering a positive mental state could support patient healing and well-being.

## The Science of Affirmations

### The Brain's Response to Positive Thinking[xii]

In nursing, positive thinking works as a vital tool for personal and professional growth. Affirmations, positive statements designed to foster self-belief and motivation, have shown potential in enhancing self-esteem and resilience among healthcare professionals.

While some may dismiss positive affirmations as pseudoscience, scientific research has begun to validate their benefits. Studies suggest that using empowering self-talk can lead to measurable improvements in well-being. Although ongoing research is needed to understand the impact of positive thinking fully, current findings are promising, particularly in fields like affective neuroscience, which explores how the brain processes emotions. This research has highlighted the significant role of both positive and negative thoughts in overall well-being.

Recent studies have also linked positive affirmations to physical and mental health benefits, improved learning, and better interpersonal relationships. By replacing negative thought patterns with healthier, more constructive ones, affirmations can positively influence the brain and body. These mantras promote positive thinking and reinforce core values, enabling nurses to respond more effectively to daily challenges.

For nurses, practicing positive affirmations can lead to increased self-confidence, a stronger sense of self-worth, and a reduction in the harmful effects of stress. This may include lower cortisol levels, the stress hormone associated with various physical and mental health issues like weight gain, sleep disturbances, and an increased risk of heart disease. By embracing positive thinking, nurses can better support their well-being, which is crucial for providing the best care to their patients.

## What Is the Science Behind Positive Affirmations?

The success of positive daily affirmations may have roots in neuroscience, which explores the structure and function of the human nervous system. By repeating affirming statements, the brain can form new neural pathways that create physical connections to these repeated thoughts.

Essentially, strengthening these pathways makes it easier for the mind to return to these positive statements and thinking patterns rather than falling back into negative thinking. Eventually, this can lead to positive mental and physical outcomes associated with self-related thoughts, such as enhanced self-esteem and confidence.

## The Science Behind Affirmations: How Effective Are They?

Research on the effectiveness of positive affirmations reveals mixed outcomes. In one study, individuals with low self-esteem who repeated positive affirmations experienced a decline in self-esteem and mood. Conversely, those with high self-esteem saw improvements in both mood and self-esteem after engaging in the same practice.

Understanding the impact of affirmations is closely tied to the concept of neuroplasticity, the brain's ability to reorganize and form new neural connections through experience and learning. Neuroimaging studies, including those using functional magnetic resonance imaging (FMRI), have shown that positive affirmations activate brain regions involved in positive emotion regulation and reward processing.

However, it is crucial to acknowledge the limitations of affirmations and their varying effects on different individuals. The same neuroimaging study affirms that the effectiveness of affirmations may depend on individual differences and the context in which they are used. Additionally, factors such as a person's mindset and the specificity of the affirmations can influence how well they work.

## The Neuroscience Behind Positive Thinking

Recent research into how the brain responds to positive and negative thinking and emotions has utilized advanced neuroimaging techniques to monitor changes in brain activity. These studies indicate that individuals with a more positive outlook—those inclined toward positive emotions—may be less reactive to emotional stimuli than negative thinkers. This affirms they may have better control over their emotional responses in stressful situations, likely because the amygdala, the brain region responsible for regulating emotions and encoding memories, is less responsive to negative stimuli in happier individuals.

Scientific evidence also supports that practices like mindfulness and various forms of meditation can influence how the brain processes emotional stimuli. For instance, individuals who engage in self-affirmation focused on future-oriented values may exhibit increased activity in brain regions associated with self-processing and valuation compared to those without.

One study demonstrated that self-affirmation could alter the brain's reward system, activating areas that link positive stimuli with positive outcomes. As a result, individuals with a positive self-image and a strong sense of self-integrity may more strongly connect positive affirmations with their desired outcomes.

The effectiveness of self-affirmation largely depends on repetition. Recent research affirms that people are likelier to believe information they hear repeatedly than statements they encounter only once. This repetition aids in self-related processing and can create an illusion of truthfulness. Repeating positive statements about oneself is more likely to be perceived as true, helping to reinforce positive thinking over negative thoughts.

Individuals may engage in various negative thinking patterns, including:

- Catastrophizing
- Overgeneralizing
- Jumping to conclusions
- All-or-nothing categorizing

These thought patterns can severely impact almost every aspect of someone's life, including health, family, education, and employment.

## Positive Thinking and Physical Health

The impact of positive thinking on physical health has been widely researched, with significant implications for the nursing profession. Positive thinking has been shown to benefit cardiovascular health, immune function, and pain perception.

For example, one study found that optimistic individuals had a lower risk of developing cardiovascular disease than those with a more pessimistic outlook. Another study demonstrated positive thinking and increased immune function, as evidenced by higher antibody production. Additionally, positive thinking has been found to reduce pain perception in individuals suffering from chronic pain.

Rooted in the New Thought movement of the 19th century, the modern self-help industry now extensively markets books and seminars on positive thinking. This concept has also gained traction in healthcare, emphasizing the importance of maintaining a positive mindset for overall health and healing. For nurses, incorporating positive thinking into patient care can be a valuable tool for supporting patients' physical and emotional well-being. Even though these claims may appear reasonable and intuitive, they are not without challenges.[xiii]

## Positive Thinking and Mental Health

Positive thinking has been associated with improved mental health outcomes, including reduced symptoms of depression and anxiety and enhanced overall psychological well-being. Research indicates that practices such as gratitude—focusing on the positive aspects of life—can lead to lower levels of depression and anxiety. Additionally, techniques like visualizing a positive future have been linked to better psychological health.

In the field of healthcare, mental health professionals have particularly embraced positive thinking. This enthusiasm has fueled a vast self-help industry comprising books, films, seminars, and branded items (such as caps and key chains) that promote New Thought and positive thinking principles. This industry often emphasizes individual coping strategies through reading and listening to materials, sometimes bypassing conventional psychotherapeutic approaches like psychodynamic, cognitive-behavioral, and humanistic therapies.

Despite the implications of self-help motivational content on healthcare and well-being, there is enough evidence across scientific disciplines to support the power of positive thinking. Positive thinking has been shown to change the brain's structure and function and improve physical and mental health outcomes. As a result, positive thinking can be a valuable tool in nursing practice, promoting positive patient outcomes and overall well-being.

# Chapter 3: Quantum Physics and the Inter-connected Web of Healing Energy!

Quantum physics, the study of the behavior of matter and energy at the atomic and subatomic level, has been a topic of fascination and scientific inquiry for over a century. Its principles have revolutionized our understanding of the nature of reality and led to a host of technological advances. Modern science demonstrates that the fundamental nature of the universe is energy. Max Planck, the father of quantum theory, famously stated: "All matter originates and exists only by a force. We must assume behind this force the existence of a conscious and intelligent Mind. This Mind is the matrix of all matter." (Planck, 1944).

This insight establishes the universe as an interconnected web of energy in which matter is not static but dynamic, flowing, and responsive to thought and observation. Quantum physics, particularly the observer effect, demonstrates that the act of observation influences the behavior of particles. This phenomenon highlights the profound relationship between consciousness and the quantum field, suggesting that human thoughts and emotions interact directly with reality's energetic matrix (Rosenblum & Kuttner, 2011).

In nursing practice, this principle can be applied to patient care by recognizing the influence of mindset and belief systems on recovery. By addressing patient's energetic and emotional needs, nurses can facilitate healing on a deeper level. For example, creating an environment that fosters positivity, gratitude, and hope amplifies the energetic coherence needed for recovery.

This chapter integrates scientific discoveries, spiritual insights, and transformative thought to explore the interconnectedness of energy, thoughts, emotions, and beliefs in shaping reality. Drawing from quantum physics, consciousness studies, and universal principles, the Quantum Nursing Theory recognizes that humans, as energetic beings, interact with an intelligent and dynamic field capable of fostering healing, transformation, and desired outcomes. By aligning thoughts and emotions with the universe's vibrational frequencies, both individuals and caregivers can activate the quantum field's potential for healing.

The new nursing theory is based on the concept that Love is the universal healing force for good health and healing. It incorporates ideas from Quantum physics, which affirms that everything in the universe is interconnected and made up of energy. Epigenetics posits that environmental factors can influence the expression of genes, and Neuroplasticity affirms that the brain is capable of changing and adapting to new experiences. However, how does quantum physics relate to the field of nursing? This chapter will explore the relationship between quantum physics and nursing practice, including the implications of quantum principles for nursing theory, research, and clinical practice.

## Quantum Physics

Quantum physics is a fundamental theory that explains natural phenomena at the atomic and subatomic levels. It encompasses the study of quantum effects like entanglement, superposition, and tunneling. This field of study has revolutionized our understanding of the physical world and led to the development of many emerging technologies, such as quantum computing, sensors, cryptography, and simulation, which have transformed our lives.

The principles of quantum physics fundamentally differ from those of classical physics, with which we are all familiar. Classical physics deals with the behavior of macroscopic objects, while quantum physics deals with the behavior of particles at the atomic and subatomic levels.

The principles of quantum physics have also found application in many areas of life, including nursing practice. In this chapter, we will explore the relationship between quantum physics and nursing practice and how the principles of quantum physics can be applied to improve the quality of nursing care.

**Quantum Mechanics**

Quantum mechanics is the basic mathematical framework that underpins it all. It was first developed in the 1920s by Niels Bohr, Werner Heisenberg, Erwin Schrödinger, and others. It characterizes simple things, such as how the position or momentum of a single particle or a group of a few particles changes over time. Both "**quantum mechanics**" and "**quantum** physics" mean the study of subatomic particles. However, "quantum mechanics" is more specific. It is the term used for the field once formulated into mathematical laws.

The principles of quantum mechanics have been used to develop many technologies in nursing practice. For example, quantum mechanics has been used to develop technologies such as magnetic resonance imaging (MRI) and positron emission tomography (PET) scanners to diagnose and treat diseases.

## Principles of Quantum Physics

Quantum physics principles are based on the idea that everything in the universe is made up of energy. This energy can be in the form of particles or waves, and it can exist in multiple states at the same time.

The following are some of the key principles of quantum physics:

1. **Superposition:** This principle states that particles can exist in multiple states simultaneously. For example, an electron can be in multiple positions around the nucleus of an atom simultaneously.
2. **Entanglement:** This principle states that particles can become entangled, meaning their properties are linked. When one particle is measured, the other particle's properties are instantly determined, even if they are far apart.
3. **Observation:** This principle states that particles do not have a definite state until they are observed. Before observation, particles exist in a probability state, meaning they can exist simultaneously in multiple states.
4. **Non-locality:** This principle states that particles can communicate with each other instantaneously, even if large distances separate them.

# An Experiment That Raises More Questions Than It Answers

The Double-Slit Experiment

**Quantum Entanglement**

*Quantum entanglement, as proposed by Einstein, Podolsky, and Rosen in 1935 and later proven by experiments such as those conducted by Alain Aspect in the 1980s, describes a situation where two or more particles become linked and instantaneously affect each other, no matter the distance separating them (Einstein et al., 1935; Aspect et al., 1982). This non-locality affirms a deep connection between particles, challenging the classical notion of separateness in the universe.*

*Probably the most famous of all is the Double-Slit experiment. The history of this experiment dates back to 1801, but at that time, it had nothing to do with quantum physics. It served as evidence for the wave nature of light. It is one of the most famous experiments in quantum physics, fundamentally challenging our understanding of reality. It reveals that the nature of reality is not fixed but rather dependent on observation and consciousness. In the experiment, photons are fired from a laser cannon through a vertical slit, and an obstacle/display is placed behind the slit on which these particles are collected and on which we see the results.*

*The experiment implies that reality does not exist in a definite state until it is observed. This challenges classical physics, which assumes the universe exists independently of observation. Some interpretations suggest that consciousness plays a role in collapsing the quantum wave function—meaning that reality as we experience it might be shaped by our awareness and perception.*

*Quantum mechanics, as demonstrated by the double-slit experiment, shows that at the subatomic level, reality operates on probabilities rather than fixed deterministic laws.*

*As we expect, the trace on the barrier is a vertical line drawn from the impact of many particles. When we add the second slot, the expected result is two vertical lines. The first logical conclusion would be that the particles interfere with each other and that after passing through the slits, they collide and spoil the result.*

*The scientists then fire one photon at a time from the laser, but the result is identical; again, we have an interference image. The only possibility for this to happen is for the photon fired from the laser cannon to pass through both slits at the same time, i.e., one particle passes through two openings! After passing, it collides with itself and leaves a mark as if it were a wave.*

*Scientists immediately wanted to investigate this shocking discovery further. How could it pass through both openings at the same time? A detector is placed to record when a photon passes through a slit. However, as soon as the detector is there, the photon again behaves as a particle, not a wave. Again, when the detector is removed, all the photons fired make an imprint as if it were a wave. How does a photon know somebody is recording it? Particles exist in multiple potential states until observed, reinforcing that the universe is not strictly mechanical but fluid and dynamic.*

*The experiment supports the idea that our perception might shape reality at the fundamental level. It raises profound questions about the nature of free will, the mind-matter connection, and the role of consciousness in the universe. Some interpretations, such as those in quantum consciousness theories, propose that the observer effect hints at a deeper, intelligent, and interconnected universe, aligning with ideas in spiritual and metaphysical traditions.*

*The double-slit experiment demonstrates that our reality is not purely physical but is influenced by observation, consciousness, and the probabilistic nature of quantum mechanics. It challenges our classical understanding of the universe and opens the door to exploring the deeper relationship between mind, matter, and the fundamental fabric of existence.*

Quantum physics provides a strong scientific basis for understanding how energy operates in the universe. Everything in the universe is made up of energy and matter, and energy is constantly flowing and interacting with matter. Quantum physics shows that particles can be interconnected and entangled, meaning they can communicate instantaneously regardless of the distance between them. The anomalous behaviors of matter at a subatomic level play a significant role in unified field theory and quantum physics, i.e., at the subatomic level, particles do not behave as separate entities but instead exhibit wave-like behavior, known as wave-particle duality.

## Applying These Concepts to Nursing Care Delivery

In nursing, these ideas can be translated into practices that enhance the care environment, improve patient outcomes, and empower nurses and patients to participate actively in healing. The underlying principle is that intentionality, imagination, and belief can influence health outcomes by directing energy and focus in meaningful ways.

Like quantum observers, nurses can influence the "field" of care through their intentionality. Before entering a patient's room, a nurse can pause to visualize the patient healing and experiencing peace. A nurse caring for a post-operative patient might focus on the intention, "This patient's body is healing perfectly, and they are comfortable and at ease." Nurses can project positive energy and thoughts into the care environment, much like shaping the probability wave in quantum physics. The use of calm tones, positive affirmations, and visualization techniques can create a harmonious atmosphere that supports recovery.

Just as the observer affects the outcome in the double-slit experiment, patients can learn to "observe" their desired health outcomes through visualization. They can educate patients to imagine themselves in a state of health vividly. A cancer patient undergoing chemotherapy can be guided to visualize their body actively fighting cancer cells and growing stronger. Patients can be encouraged to adopt affirmations that align with their health goals, helping them shift their focus from fear or doubt to positive expectations. A patient with chronic pain might repeat affirmations such as, "My body is strong, and I feel better every day."

When nurses intentionally foster trust and connection, they create a collaborative healing environment. A nurse could use Goddard-inspired techniques to assume the feeling of a positive interaction with a patient, visualizing the patient feeling safe, understood, and supported. Incorporating Imogene King's Theory of Goal Attainment, nurses and patients can collaboratively visualize desired outcomes, aligning their intentions for recovery. For example, nurses and patients might sit together and visualize the patient walking independently after a physical therapy session.

Neville Goddard's teachings on intention and imagination, the observer effect in quantum physics, and the findings of the double-slit experiment collectively emphasize the power of consciousness to shape outcomes. In nursing, this can translate into a deliberate focus on positive intention, visualization, and belief as integral components of care delivery and patient education. By harnessing these principles, nurses and patients can collaboratively influence health outcomes, creating a deeply interconnected and holistic approach to healing.

## The Non-Locality of the Physical Reality

Classical physics posits that physical reality is inherently local, meaning that an event or measurement at one point in space cannot influence another event occurring at a distant location beyond a relatively short range. This principle was long regarded as an unalterable law of nature. However, in 1997, experiments were conducted in which light particles (photons) were generated under specific conditions and traveled in opposite directions to detectors approximately seven miles apart. Remarkably, the results demonstrated that the photons "interacted" or "communicated" with one another instantaneously, challenging the notion of locality. This groundbreaking discovery revealed that physical reality is, in fact, non-local, a finding that Robert Nadeau and Menas Kafatos describe as one of the most significant in the history of science.

In support of their transformative argument, the authors trace the fascinating historical developments that led to the discovery of non-locality and the intense debates among the scientists responsible for these breakthroughs. Ultimately, the authors contend that this new understanding affirms a closer relationship between mind and nature than previously conceived. Their work presents a revolutionary exploration of the profound implications of non-locality, particularly its impact on the fundamental human experience of consciousness.

## Dr. Masaru Emoto's Work in the Context of Quantum Physics and Entanglement

The relationship between consciousness and physical reality has intrigued scientists and philosophers for centuries. Dr. Masaru Emoto's research on water crystals and the influence of human thought can be related to concepts in quantum physics, particularly the theory of entanglement. Quantum entanglement, a phenomenon where particles remain interconnected regardless of distance, affirms that the universe is more connected at a fundamental level than classical physics allows.

Dr. Emoto's ideas intersect with quantum entanglement and their implications for understanding the power of thought and healing. The implications of entanglement extend beyond the subatomic world. Some theorists have posited that entanglement might be a feature of consciousness itself, potentially offering a scientific basis for phenomena such as telepathy, collective consciousness, or the influence of thought on physical reality (Penrose, 1994).

Dr. Emoto suggested that thoughts and emotions could influence the molecular structure of water, leading to different crystalline forms when frozen. This affirms a possible connection between human consciousness and the physical world, echoing the principles of quantum entanglement.

Following Dr. Masaru Emoto's work, experiments were conducted using containers of cooked rice. Groups directed different emotions or intentions (positive, negative, neutral) toward the rice. The rice exposed to loving thoughts or gratitude decomposed more slowly; however, the rice exposed to hateful or negative thoughts showed signs of rapid decay. This suggests that collective focus and emotional intention can influence the physical state of organic matter.

## The Power of Thought and Healing

Research in psychoneuroimmunology has demonstrated that positive mental states can enhance immune function and promote quicker recovery from illness (Pert, 1999). Although, these outcomes are commonly attributed to biochemical mechanisms, quantum entanglement offers a potential framework for understanding how thought and consciousness may directly influence physiological processes (Schwartz et al., 2005).

The intersection of Emoto's findings and quantum physics provides an avenue for investigating the role of thoughts in healing. Quantum entanglement, which posits that the connection between entangled particles is unaffected by spatial distance, may likewise extend to the impact of positive thoughts or intentions on an individual's health, regardless of physical proximity (Dossey, 2014).

## Applying Quantum Physics Principles in Nursing Practice

The principles of quantum physics have significant implications for nursing practice. Nurses could use them to improve patient care and promote healing. The following are some ways that quantum physics principles could be applied in nursing practice:

1. **Holistic Care:** The principles of quantum physics suggest that everything in the universe is interconnected. This means that the mind, body, and spirit are all connected, and treating one without considering the others is incomplete. Nurses who understand this can provide holistic care that addresses their patients' physical, emotional, and spiritual needs.
2. **Energy Healing:** The principles of quantum physics suggest that everything comprises energy. Nurses can use this understanding to provide energy healing, which involves manipulating patients' energy fields to promote healing. Techniques such as Reiki and therapeutic touch are based on quantum physics.
3. **Mind-Body Connection:** The principles of quantum physics suggest that the mind and body are interconnected. Nurses can use this understanding to help patients improve their health by promoting positive thinking, stress reduction, and other mind-body techniques.
4. **Patient-Centered Care:** The principles of quantum physics suggest that everything is connected, including the patient and their environment. Nurses can use this understanding to provide patient-centered care, considering the patient's needs and preferences.
5. **Telehealth:** The principles of quantum physics suggest that particles can communicate with each other instantly, even if large distances separate them. Nurses can use this understanding to provide tele-health services, such as video conferencing and remote monitoring, to communicate with patients and other healthcare providers in real-time.
6. **Preventative Care:** The principles of quantum physics suggest that particles exist in a state of probability until they are observed. Nurses can use this understanding to

provide preventative care that addresses potential health problems before they become severe.
7. **Interdisciplinary Collaboration:** The principles of quantum physics suggest that everything is interconnected. Nurses can use this understanding to collaborate with other healthcare providers, such as physicians, therapists, and social workers, to provide comprehensive care that addresses all aspects of the patient's health.

The potential implications of quantum entanglement in nursing and healthcare are profound. If consciousness can influence physical reality, as suggested by quantum theories and Emoto's work, healthcare providers' attitudes, intentions, and mental states could directly impact patient outcomes. This perspective encourages a holistic approach to care, where patients' and caregivers' mental and emotional states are considered integral to the healing process (Benor, 2001).

Moreover, understanding these concepts could lead to developing new therapeutic modalities that leverage the power of positive thought and intentionality, much like practices in energy medicine and holistic nursing (Jonas & Crawford, 2003). Integrating quantum principles into nursing education could also foster a deeper understanding of the interconnectedness of mind and body, enhancing patient care through a more comprehensive approach to healing.

Quantum entanglement provides a compelling framework for understanding the nurse-patient relationship. In traditional nursing models, the relationship between the nurse and the patient is seen as a therapeutic alliance that can majorly impact health outcomes. Quantum entanglement affirms that this connection is more profound than previously understood. Just as entangled particles influence each other instantaneously, a nurse's thoughts, emotions, and intentions directly impact the patient's health (Benor, 2001).

This perspective aligns with therapeutic presence in nursing, where the nurse's focused attention, empathy, and compassion are believed to facilitate healing (Kearney, 2009). If quantum entanglement plays a role in this process, it underscores the importance of the nurse's mental and emotional state in patient's care. Nurses who cultivate positive intentions and mindfulness enhance the healing process not only through their actions but also through the subtle, energetic connections they share with their patients.

Holistic nursing care is an approach to nursing care that considers the physical, emotional, social, and spiritual needs of the patient. It focuses on the whole person rather than just the disease or illness. Quantum Physics has been used to develop many holistic nursing care practices. The principles of quantum physics have implications for all aspects of nursing practices, from assessment and diagnosis to treatment and care. Quantum principles suggest that the mind and body are interconnected, and that health and well-being are not just the result of biological function but are influenced by a range of physical, emotional, social, and spiritual factors. This affirms that nurses must take a holistic approach to patient care, considering the physical symptoms of illness and the patient's beliefs, values, and lifestyle factors.

One of the principles of quantum physics applied to holistic nursing care is the principle of entanglement. Entanglement is a phenomenon where two particles are connected together in such a way that the state of one particle is dependent on the state of the other. This principle has been applied to holistic nursing care by recognizing that the state of a patient is linked to the state of the nurse caring for the patient. Therefore, it is crucial for the nurse to be in a positive and healing state of mind when caring for the patient.

Another principle of quantum physics that has been applied to holistic nursing care is the principle of superposition. Superposition is a phenomenon where a particle can exist in multiple states simultaneously. This principle has been applied to holistic nursing care by recognizing that the patient can exist in multiple states of being at the same time. Therefore, the nurses should be able to see the patients in multiple states and respond appropriately to each state. It's a crucial responsibility that requires great vigilance.

**Quantum Physics and Healing**

Quantum physics has been used to develop many healing practices. One of the principles of quantum physics applied to healing is the principle of non-locality. Non-locality is a phenomenon where two particles can be linked together in a way that one particle is dependent on other particle, even if a considerable distance separates the particles.

This principle has been applied to healing by recognizing that the healer's state is linked to the patient's state, even if a significant distance separates the healer and the patient. This has led to developing practices such as distance healing or Reiki, where the healer can send healing energy to the patient.

The principles of quantum physics have the potential to transform our understanding of health and healing, and their impact on nursing theory cannot be overstated. The traditional biomedical model of disease has been challenged by the recognition that illness is not just the result of biological dysfunction but is a complex interplay of physical, emotional, social, and spiritual factors. Quantum physics provides a framework for understanding the interconnectedness of these factors and their role in health and healing.

## The Paradigm Shift in Healthcare

Traditional healthcare has primarily been grounded in the Newtonian-Cartesian model, which views the body as a machine composed of separate parts that can be analyzed and treated independently. However, quantum physics challenges this reductionist view, suggesting that the body is a dynamic system of interconnected energy fields that interact with the environment (Capra, 1982).

This paradigm shift has significant nursing implications, and nurses have increasingly embraced a holistic approach to care. Nursing theories such as Martha Rogers' Science of Unitary Human Beings and Jean Watson's Theory of Human Caring emphasize the interconnectedness of the human being's physical, mental, and spiritual aspects (Rogers, 1970; Watson, 1979). Integrating quantum principles into nursing encourages a more deeper insight of human health, where the mind, body, and environment are seen as interrelated components of a single system.

## Quantum Physics and Nursing Research

The principles of quantum physics also have significant implications for nursing research. The traditional paradigm of randomized controlled trials, in which a single variable is isolated and tested, is unsuited for studying complex interventions involving multiple factors and interactions. Quantum principles provide a framework for understanding the complex interplay of physical, emotional, social, and spiritual factors that contribute to health and healing. It also suggests that new research methods fit appropriately in exploring these interactions completely .

Quantum physics has also been used to explain the mechanisms underlying the placebo effect, which has important implications for nursing research. Placebo-controlled trials are the gold standard for testing the efficacy of new treatments, but the placebo effect can be a confounding factor that undermines the validity of these trials. Understanding the mechanisms underlying the placebo effect can help researchers design more effective trials. It can lead to the development of new treatments that harness the power of the mind-body connection.

The Power of Mind, Love, and Holistic Health proposes that a universal force of love is present in all living beings and is responsible for maintaining health and well-being. This force is analogous to the unified force that governs the behavior of all particles in the universe. Just as the unified force is responsible for the behavior of subatomic particles, the universal force of love is responsible for the health and well-being of all living beings. The theory proposes that this force can be harnessed through practices such as meditation, Reiki, and other energy-healing modalities to promote healing and well-being.

In summary, the anomalous behaviors of matter at a subatomic level are fundamental to quantum physics. These behaviors can be explained by the presence of a single underlying force that governs the behavior of all particles in the universe.

## The Unified Field Theory and What Heals

The unified field, a concept explored by theoretical physicists such as Albert Einstein and John Hagelin, posits that all forces in the universe are interconnected at a fundamental level (Hagelin,1987). This energetic field is dynamic, intelligent, and responsive. According to Gregg Braden, this matrix acts as a "container, bridge, and mirror" for human consciousness, reflecting the energy of thoughts, emotions, and beliefs (Braden, 2007).

We primarily communicate with this field through our emotions and feelings. Emotions, as energy in motion, generate vibrational frequencies interacting with the field. Beliefs, in turn, guide these emotional signals, shaping the outcomes we experience. For instance, positive emotions like love, gratitude, and joy resonate with high frequencies that align with coherence and healing. In contrast, negative emotions such as fear and anger produce discordant vibrations that may perpetuate illness or stagnation (McCraty et al., 2009).

An example of this principle in action can be seen in patients practicing gratitude journaling. Patients often report improved mental health and a sense of well-being by focusing on positive outcomes and expressing gratitude. This practice demonstrates how emotions and beliefs shape the energetic patterns contributing to recovery and transformation.

The various energy forces described above include Chi, Reiki, Karma, and the quantum field. These are all manifestations of the universal force of love central to the Unified Field Theory. This New Nursing theory posits that everything in the universe is interconnected and that an underlying energy field permeates all creation. This energy is often described as a field of love and is believed to be the foundation of all existence.

Mindfulness meditation, which has been shown to reduce stress and improve immune function, can be seen as a way of harmonizing the individual's energy with the broader consciousness field (Shapiro, Schwartz, & Bonner, 1998). Energy healing practices like Reiki and Therapeutic Touch work on the principle that the practitioner can channel healing energy from the Unified Field into the patient, promoting healing by restoring energetic balance (Krieger, 1993).

According to the unified field theory, all the fundamental forces of nature, such as electromagnetism, weak nuclear force, strong nuclear force, and gravity, are unified at the subatomic level. The unified field theory affirms that there is a single underlying force that governs the behavior of all particles in the universe.

The concept of a Unified Field, where all forces and particles manifest a single underlying reality, has profound implications for self-healing. If the body and mind are part of a unified field, then healing would involve aligning oneself with this field to restore balance and harmony. This idea resonates with various holistic health practices, such as meditation, energy healing, and integrative medicine, which aim to tap into the body's innate healing abilities by fostering a connection with the broader field of consciousness (Dossey, 2014).

In nursing, this perspective encourages a shift from treating symptoms to addressing the underlying imbalances in the patient's energy field. Practices such as Reiki, Therapeutic Touch, and mindfulness-based stress reduction (MBSR) can be seen as ways of aligning the patient with the Unified Field, promoting self-healing by restoring the natural flow of energy (Krieger, 1993; Kabat-Zinn, 2003). Nurses trained in these modalities can offer patients an additional dimension of care beyond physical interventions, addressing the emotional, mental, and spiritual aspects of healing.

The Unified Field Theory can explain the anomalous behaviors of matter at a subatomic level, such as wave-particle duality and quantum entanglement. For example, quantum entanglement refers to the phenomenon where two particles become entangled and share a correlation independent of their distance. According to the unified field theory, this correlation occurs as the two particles are interconnected by the underlying force that governs the behavior of all particles in the universe.

The Unified Field Theory is a proposed scientific theory that aims to unify all of nature's fundamental forces, including gravity, electromagnetism, and the strong and weak nuclear forces, into a single framework. This theory postulates the existence of an essential force that permeates the entire universe, connecting all matter and energy in a seamless web of interconnectedness. This force is often called the unified field or the field of all possibilities.

The unified field concept is closely related to the universal force of love central to The Greater New Nursing Theory, i.e., The Power of Love. This theory postulates that there is a fundamental force of love that permeates the entire universe, connecting all living beings and the natural world in a seamless web of interconnectedness. This force is believed to be the source of healing, transformation, and growth, and the driving force behind all of the phenomena we observe in the world around us.

The main idea of quantum physics is that the particles are in a state of superposition, meaning that they exist in multiple states simultaneously. This is similar to the concept of the unified field, which tends to contain all possible states of existence. At the same time, the unified field is also described as a field of pure consciousness, which can be equated with the universal force of love.

From a scientific perspective, the unified field and the universal force of love can be seen as different expressions of the same underlying reality. The unified field is the field of all possibilities, the source of all energy and matter, and the fundamental fabric of the universe. The universal force of love connects all living beings, natural world phenomenon and everything that underlies in the processes of growth, transformation, and healing that we observe in the world around us. Both concepts are based on the idea that there is a fundamental interconnectedness in the universe and that all phenomena arise from this interconnectedness.

At a subatomic level, matter's behavior is anomalous and often seems to defy classical physics. This can be seen as evidence of a unified field that underlies all of the phenomena we observe in the universe. The properties of subatomic particles, such as their spin and charge, are intimately connected to the properties of the unified field and cannot be understood in isolation.

Similarly, the universal force of love is believed to underlie all the growth, transformation, and healing processes we observe in the world around us. It is the force that connects all living beings and the natural world and allows us to tap into the field of all possibilities to create the reality that we desire. By understanding the fundamental interconnectedness of all things and harnessing the power of the universal force of love, we can create a more harmonious, peaceful, and loving world.

Furthermore, the connection between the unified field theory and nursing has significant implications for the future of healthcare. As we continue to advance our understanding of quantum physics and the nature of the universe, we may discover new technologies or treatment modalities that have previously been unexplored. For example, research in quantum biology has shown that quantum phenomena play a role in cellular processes, which could have implications for the development of new treatments for disease. As nurses are at the forefront of healthcare delivery, it is essential for them to stay informed about these advancements and be prepared to incorporate new knowledge into their practice.

In conclusion, the unified field and the universal force of love are two sides of the same coin, representing the fundamental interconnectedness of all things. By understanding the relationship between these two concepts, we can gain a deeper appreciation of the underlying unity of the universe and tap into the transformative power of the universal force of love. The relationship between the unified field theory, the universal force of love, and energy forces such as Chi and Reiki have significant implications for nursing practice. By understanding these concepts, nurses can provide more comprehensive and effective patient care based on a holistic understanding of health and wellness. Furthermore, staying informed about advancements in quantum physics and related fields is essential for ensuring that nursing practice remains at the forefront of healthcare delivery.

## Integrating Quantum Principles into Clinical Practice

Integrating quantum principles into clinical practice involves applying the concepts of energy, interconnectedness, and intention to patient care. For instance, understanding that all matter and energy are interconnected can help nurses appreciate the impact of their own presence and intention on patient's outcomes. Quantum entanglement affirms that interactions between the nurses and patient are not just superficial but may involve deeper, energetically significant connections (Benor, 2001).

Practices such as mindfulness, meditation, and energy healing align with the principles of quantum physics. Mindfulness-based interventions, for example, have a proven record to reduce stress, improve emotional regulation, and enhance overall health (Kabat-Zinn, 2003). These practices can be integrated into nursing care to help patients manage chronic conditions, reduce anxiety, and improve quality of life. By focusing on the energy and intention behind their actions, nurses can create a more supportive and healing environment for their patients.

One of the core challenges faced in applying quantum principles to nursing practice is bridging the gap between scientific theory and clinical practice. While quantum physics offers exciting possibilities, it is essential to ground these ideas in practical, evidence-based research that can be applied in real-world settings. Collaborative efforts between researchers, clinicians, and educators can help translate quantum principles into actionable interventions and care practices (Dossey & Keegan, 2009).

Nursing research and quantum principles together should explore how these concepts can enhance patient care and improve health outcomes. This includes investigating the impact of mindfulness and energy-based practices on various health conditions and examining the role of the nurse-patient relationship in promoting healing (Benor, 2001; Radin, 2006).

Quantum physics challenges traditional biomedical models and offers new insights into the nature of health and healing. Unified Field Theory provides a framework for understanding the interconnectedness of all aspects of reality, including the mind, body, and spirit. By incorporating these concepts into nursing practice, education, and research, we can develop a more integrated approach to healthcare that honors the complexity and unity of human experience.

While all the challenges must be addressed, including the need for rigorous research and bridging gaps between science and practice, there are potential benefits of integrating quantum principles into nursing. By fostering a deeper understanding of the interconnected nature of health and embracing innovative approaches to care, nurses can enhance their practice and improve patient health outcomes.

## Quantum Reality, Universal Love, and Nursing Theory

The concept of a universal love force, described by Rhonda Byrne in her works "The Power" and "The Secret," presents a vision of reality where positive thinking, love, and intention shape our lives and influence our surroundings. Though rooted in popular self-help culture, Byrne's ideas intersect intriguingly with the principles of quantum mechanics and the unified field theory. This intersection becomes particularly relevant when considering the implications of quantum reality for nursing theory, especially in the context of Martha Rogers' Science of Unitary Human Beings. Rogers' theory posits that humans are energy fields constantly interacting with their environments. This idea aligns with quantum theory and Byrne's notion of a universal love force.

While Byrne's ideas have been widely popularized and embraced by many, they also align with certain principles of quantum mechanics, particularly the idea that consciousness and intention can influence the physical world. The concept of a universal love force resonates with the quantum view of the universe as a unified field of interconnected energy, where everything is fundamentally connected and influenced by the forces of consciousness and intention.

Rogers' theory is built upon five key assumptions:

- **Wholeness**: Human beings are viewed as complete, indivisible entities that cannot be understood by simply analyzing their parts.
- **Openness**: Human beings and their environments are open systems that continuously exchange energy and information.
- **Pattern**: The pattern of an individual's energy field is unique and reflects the complex interactions between the person and their environment.
- **Pan-dimensionality**: Human beings exist in a pan-dimensional reality, where time, space, and other dimensions are fluid and interconnected.
- **Resonance**: Human interaction with their environments is characterized by rhythmic, harmonious energy exchanges.

The principles of quantum mechanics, particularly quantum entanglement, resonate deeply with the foundational concepts of Rogers' Science of Unitary Human Beings. Both frameworks reject reductionism in favor of a holistic view that emphasizes the interconnectedness of all things. In Rogers' theory, human beings are seen as unitary energy fields, constantly interacting with their environments in a dynamic, non-linear fashion. This view aligns with the quantum reality proposed by Zeilinger's work, where particles are not isolated entities but are instead part of a larger, interconnected whole.

## Future Implications for Nursing Theory

Integrating quantum principles, the unified field theory, and the concept of a universal love force into nursing theory offers exciting possibilities for the future of healthcare. By embracing these ideas, future nursing theories can provide a more comprehensive understanding of health and healing, transcending the limitations of classical, reductionist models.

1. **Advancing Holistic Nursing**: Incorporating universal love and quantum principles into nursing theory supports the advancement of holistic nursing, where care is centered on the whole person, including their physical, mental, emotional, and spiritual dimensions. This approach encourages nurses to develop practices that nurture all aspects of a patient's well-being, recognizing the interconnected nature of health.
2. **Research and Evidence-Based Practice**: As the integration of quantum principles and universal love into nursing theory progresses, there is a growing need for research to explore the effectiveness of these ideas in clinical practice. Studies could examine the impact of positive intention, therapeutic presence, and holistic care

on patient outcomes, contributing to the development of evidence-based practices that align with these concepts.
3. **Education and Training**: To fully integrate these ideas into nursing practice, education and training programs must be developed that teach nurses about the principles of quantum mechanics, the unified field theory, and the power of love and intention in healing. By equipping nurses with this knowledge, we can foster a new generation of healthcare providers prepared to deliver care that aligns with these advanced theoretical concepts.
4. **Global Health and Social Justice**: The interconnectedness emphasized by quantum entanglement and the universal love force has implications for global health and social justice. Future nursing theories could explore how these concepts can inform efforts to address health disparities, promote social equity, and improve the overall well-being of populations worldwide.
5. **Spiritual Care and Mindfulness**: Integrating quantum principles and universal love into nursing theory also supports the inclusion of spiritual care and mindfulness practices in healthcare. These practices align with the principles of interconnectedness and positive intention and help patients achieve greater balance and harmony in their lives, supporting their overall health and well-being.

Martha Rogers' Science of Unitary Human Beings challenges reductionist approaches to patient care, advocating for a holistic perspective that recognizes the dynamic interactions between individuals and their surroundings. Integrating the concept of a universal love force, as described by Rhonda Byrne, into nursing theory can further enhance our understanding of health and healing. This integration supports the development of future nursing theories that embrace holistic, patient-centered care and recognize the profound impact of love, intention, and consciousness on the healing process.

As we continue to explore the implications of quantum mechanics, the unified field theory, and universal love for nursing theory, we must approach these ideas with enthusiasm and scientific rigor. The potential to enhance patient care and deepen our understanding of health and healing is immense. Still, it is crucial to ensure that these practices are grounded in evidence and delivered in an ethical, safe, and effective way.

The intersection of quantum reality, universal love, and nursing theory represents a promising new healthcare direction that aligns scientific advancements with holistic, patient-centered care. By embracing these principles, nursing can continue to evolve as a discipline that recognizes the unity and interconnectedness of all things, promoting health and healing in a way that honors human beings' complexity and wholeness.

In conclusion, the concept of life force energy has been recognized across many cultures and spiritual traditions. While modern science has slowly acknowledged its existence, recent quantum physics discoveries demonstrate a scientific basis for this phenomenon. From a spiritual and metaphysical perspective, the life force energy is the essence of the divine that animates all living things, connecting us to the larger universe. By understanding and harnessing this energy, we can promote physical, emotional, and spiritual well-being and deepen our connection to the fundamental unity of all things.

# References

Quantum Physics: Encyclopedia of Condensed Matter Physics (Second Edition), 2024. Read at: https://www.sciencedirect.com/topics/physics-and-astronomy/quantum-physics

Quantum Physics by Richard Webb. Read at: https://www.newscientist.com/definition/quantum-physics/

What is the difference between quantum mechanics and quantum physics? Quantum Physics Lady: Encyclopedia Of Quantum Physics And Consciousness. Read here.

Nadeau, R., & Kafatos, M. (2001). *The Non-Local Universe: The New Physics and Matters of the Mind*. Oxford University Press.

Nevena Glogovac. (2023). *The Strangely Fascinating World Of Quantum Physics. Read Here.*

Benor, D. J. (2001). *Spiritual Healing: Scientific Validation of a Healing Revolution*. Vision Publications.

Dossey, L. (2014). *One Mind: How Our Individual Mind Is Part of a Greater Consciousness and Why It Matters*. Hay House.

Jonas, W. B., & Crawford, C. C. (2003). *Healing, Intention, and Energy Medicine: Science, Research Methods, and Clinical Implications*. Churchill Livingstone.

Penrose, R. (1994). *Shadows of the Mind: A Search for the Missing Science of Consciousness*. Oxford University Press.

Pert, C. B. (1999). *Molecules of Emotion: The Science Behind Mind-Body Medicine*. Simon & Schuster.

Schwartz, G. E., Russek, L. G., & Simon, W. L. (2005). *The Living Energy Universe: A Fundamental Discovery That Transforms Science and Medicine*. Hampton Roads Publishing

Benor, D. J. (2001). *Spiritual Healing: Scientific Validation of a Healing Revolution*. Vision Publications.

Capra, F. (1982). *The Tao of Physics: An Exploration of the Parallels Between Modern Physics and Eastern Mysticism*. Shambhala Publications.

Dossey, L. (2008). *The Science of Premonitions: How Knowing the Future Can Shape Our Lives*. Harmony Books.

Kearney, M. (2009). *The Therapeutic Use of Self in Nursing: Developing the Skills of Therapeutic Presence*. Springer Publishing Company.

Radin, D. (2006). *Entangled Minds: Extrasensory Experiences in a Quantum Reality*. Paraview Pocket Books.

# Chapter 4: The Power of Intention and Visualization

## Overview

Our thoughts, emotions, and intentions are all forms of energy that can influence our physical world. Intentions and Visualization shape our reality. When our thoughts take the form of an intention, they set the manifestation in motion, which, if visualized in the best of detail, forms our reality, positive or negative. Is it that simple? If you comprehend the world and its secrets in energies, frequencies, and vibrations, you can paraphrase Nikola Tesla.

Whether the thoughts are positive or negative, intrusive or instructive, objective or subjective, they carry measurable energy that can affect the world around us. Gregg Braden, a renowned author and scientist, explored the connection between prayer, consciousness, and quantum physics. In his book, 'The Divine Matrix: Bridging Time, Space, Miracles, and Belief,' he highlights how our thoughts and emotions influence the world around us and how we can harness the power of consciousness to create positive change. Quantum science now reveals that our thoughts and emotions are not just abstract concepts but measurable energy that can tremendously affect the world around us.

"Quantum physics looks at the universe differently. In recent years, scientists have developed the technology that has made it possible to document the strange and sometimes miraculous behavior of quantum energy that forms the essence of the universe and our bodies. For example, quantum energy can exist in two different forms: visible particles or invisible waves. Either way, the energy is still there, making itself known in different forms.

Quantum particles can communicate with themselves at different points in time. The concepts of past, present, and future do not limit them. To a quantum particle, this is now, and there is here."

According to Braden, prayer is not just a religious practice but a scientifically proven technique that can change the world around us. He explains that our thoughts and intentions directly impact the energy around us, and when we pray, we tap into the divine matrix and amplify our intentions. This aligns with the quantum nursing theory's principle that energy is never created or destroyed but is always moving.

One way prayer affects reality on a subatomic level is through the power of intention. Intention is the focused and directed use of the mind to create a desired outcome. Research has shown that intention can have a measurable effect on physical systems, including the behavior of subatomic particles.

The Maharishi Effect is based on studies where groups practicing Transcendental Meditation were shown to influence societal outcomes like crime rates, violence, and economic conditions. In one experiment, a large group of meditators was gathered in Washington, D.C., in 1993 to meditate to reduce violent crime. Crime rates reportedly dropped by 23% during the meditation, dissipating the effect afterward. This suggests that collective thought, like a prayer in the congregation or a meditation, in this case, particularly focused on peace and positive intentions, can have observable effects on societal dynamics.

Studies have also examined the effects of collective prayer or intention on health outcomes. One such study involved distant prayer for patients in an intensive care unit (ICU). Patients who were the focus of intentional prayer often showed better recovery rates, reduced complications, and shorter hospital stays than those who were not.

Collective prayer or focused intention affects healing processes, even when the recipient is unaware of the prayer.

In nursing, this means that we can utilize our thoughts, emotions, and beliefs to manifest the outcomes we want for our patients and ourselves. For instance, if we create a healing environment for our patients, we can cultivate feelings of love, compassion, and gratitude and focus our thoughts on the positive outcomes we want. Doing so sends a powerful signal to the unified field of love that attracts the frequencies and vibrations that align with our intentions.

Braden's work also aligns with the principles of the New Nursing Theory, which emphasizes the role of positive thought, intention, and love-based emotions in healing. The theory proposes that by cultivating mindfulness, we can tap into the quantum field and access a range of potentials that can influence our health and well-being.

Moreover, it emphasizes the importance of intention and focused attention in healthcare. By directing positive intentions and attention toward patients, nurses can potentially influence their patients' energy fields, promoting healing and well-being. This concept is supported by research in mind-body medicine, which has demonstrated the power of intention and attention in promoting healing and positive health outcomes (Dossey, 2013).

The New Nursing Theory proposed in this book accentuates that energetic and electromagnetic existence is the truth of our existence, which has been vastly overlooked and underutilized in past endeavors when applying effort and intent to healthcare.

# What is Intention?

**Britannica** defines **Intention** as (Latin: intentio), which, in scholastic logic and psychology, is a concept used to describe a mode of being or relation. In knowing, the mind is said to "intend" or "tend toward" its object, and a thing as known, or in the knowing mind, has "intentional being". Intention would mean either the mind knowing or the knowledge itself, analogous to the use of perception for the act of perceiving or the thing perceived. The first intention is knowledge of a thing in itself; the second intention is knowledge of the thing as known. Thus, the term man is in first intention in the statement "man is mortal," but in second intention in "man is a species." Logic was held by the scholastics to consist of the study of second intentions.

## McTaggart, L - The Intention Experiment

Since 2007, Lynne has collaborated with teams of scientists from prestigious universities and engaged thousands of international readers across more than 100 countries, creating the world's largest "global laboratory" to conduct some of the earliest controlled experiments on the power of mass intention. At various intervals, she invites her audience to direct a specific thought toward a designated target, after which the scientific teams analyze the results to assess any observable changes.

Of Lynne's 39 experiments thus far, 35 have demonstrated positive, measurable, and, in many cases, statistically significant effects. These experiments have indicated that collective intention can alter the subtle properties of plants, accelerate seed growth, purify water, reduce violence in conflict zones or deprived areas, and even contribute to the healing of patients suffering from severe PTSD. However, the most profound impact of group intention is the transformative experience it creates for the participants, fostering a deep sense of unity.

For instance, following peace Intention Experiments, participants report feeling more peaceful and loving in their own lives, while healing experiments often result in the participants experiencing personal healing. Thousands of individuals who have participated in Lynne's Intention Experiments have reported recovering from chronic health conditions, repairing relationships, discovering a renewed sense of purpose, or transitioning from routine jobs to more fulfilling careers.

The Intention Experiment details the work physicians, physicists, and consciousness researchers have done since then to reveal how inextricably intertwined mind and matter really are. This uplifting and empowering vision of human potential heals the Cartesian split between mind and matter. It provides evidence that humans form a single concrescence with each other and the world around us.

## Dr. Masaru Emoto's Water Studies

Dr. Masaru Emoto's water studies have gained significant attention in the fields of alternative and holistic medicine, spirituality, and environmentalism. Emoto's work is based on the concept that water is capable of storing and transmitting information and that human thoughts, words, and emotions can influence the molecular structure of water. Emoto's research has profound implications for nursing practice, particularly in patient-centered care, therapeutic communication, and environmental health.

Emoto's water studies involved exposing water samples to various stimuli, such as music, words, and thoughts, and then freezing them to examine their crystal structures under a microscope. Emoto claimed that water exposed to positive stimuli, such as classical music or loving words, formed beautiful, symmetrical crystal structures, while water exposed to negative stimuli, such as heavy metal music or hateful words, formed chaotic and irregular crystal structures. Although Emoto's methodology and interpretation of results have been criticized by some scientists, his work has sparked interest and discussion about the nature of water and the power of human intention.

One of the most relevant and relatable parts of Emoto's work to nursing practice is the idea that human thoughts, words, and emotions can influence the molecular structure of water. This concept has significant implications for nurses to communicate with patients and create healing environments. Therapeutic communication involves listening attentively, using empathic responses, and conveying positive messages, creating a positive emotional atmosphere that would enhance the patient's healing process. Similarly, creating a healing environment that is calming, comfortable, and aesthetically pleasing can positively impact the patient's emotional and physical well-being.

Additionally, Emoto's work has implications for environmental health, as water is an essential component of the natural world and the human body. Nurses can promote ecological health by advocating for policies that protect water resources, educating patients and families about the importance of clean water, and incorporating environmentally sustainable practices into healthcare settings.

**Case Study 1:**

Mrs. J is a 60-year-old woman who was recently diagnosed with breast cancer. She is scheduled for surgery next week and is feeling anxious and overwhelmed. Mrs. J expresses her fears and concerns about the surgery and recovery during her preoperative visit with the nurse. The nurse listens attentively and uses empathic responses to validate Mrs. J's feelings. The nurse also shares positive messages, such as "You are strong and resilient, and I believe you will recover quickly." After the visit, the nurse decorates Mrs. J's room with flowers and calming artwork to create a healing environment. Mrs. J reports feeling more relaxed and optimistic about her surgery.

**Case Study 2:**

Mr. S is a 45-year-old man who was admitted to the hospital with pneumonia. During his stay, he complained about the hospital's tap water, which he found unpleasant to drink. The nurse explained to Mr. S the importance of staying hydrated for his recovery and offered him bottled water. The nurse also educates Mr. S about the hospital's water treatment processes and the importance of clean water for health. Mr. S reports feeling more comfortable drinking bottled water and expresses gratitude for the nurse's efforts to improve his hospital experience.

## In the Context of Nursing:

As nurses, we have the power to influence the energy field of our patients through our thoughts, emotions, and intentions. By understanding the interconnectedness of all things and the power of intention and energy, nurses can create a healing environment that supports the patient's physical, emotional, and spiritual needs.

By understanding the power of intention, energy, and interconnectedness, nurses can create a healing environment that supports the patient's physical, emotional, and spiritual needs. This can lead to improved outcomes, reduced stress and anxiety, and an overall well-being for both the patient and the nurse. Another way to communicate with the unified field of love is through visualization and intention. By creating a clear mental picture of what we want to manifest and holding that image in our minds, we send a powerful signal to the field that we are ready and willing to receive our desired outcome. This can be especially effective when combined with positive affirmations and a strong belief in the power of the field.

We will also examine the practical implications of these theories for nursing practice. For example, we will explore the role of consciousness and intentionality in promoting healing and well-being and how nurses can leverage these concepts to enhance patient outcomes. We will also examine the challenges of integrating quantum physics and the unified field theory into nursing practice. These may include resistance from patients or healthcare providers unfamiliar with these concepts, as well as the need for additional education and training.

Finally, we will provide practical strategies for integrating quantum physics and the unified field theory into nursing practice. These may include incorporating meditation or visualization techniques into patient care or using intentionality to promote healing and well-being. We will explore how positive thinking can be applied to nursing practice. We will examine how nurses can promote positive thinking in their patients through the use of affirmations, visualization, and other techniques. We will also explore how nurses can cultivate positive thinking in themselves, even in challenging or stressful situations. Finally, we will provide practical strategies for promoting positive thinking in nursing practice. These could include incorporating mindfulness practices into patient care, using positive self-talk and visualization techniques, and providing patients with resources and support to help them cultivate a positive mindset.

We will examine a case study of a patient who was suffering from chronic pain and depression. The patient had been receiving conventional medical treatments for years but had seen slight improvement. With the support of their nurse, the patient began incorporating positive thinking and visualization techniques into their daily routine. Over time, the patient's pain and depression began to improve, and they were able to reduce their reliance on medication. This can be done through affirmations, visualizations, and other techniques that promote positive thinking.

## What is Visualization & Imagery?

The concept of visualization, a central tenet of New Thought philosophy, has found practical application in nursing practice. Visualization involves mentally envisioning oneself in a particular scenario and experiencing it with heightened vividness. Empirical studies have demonstrated the efficacy of visualization as a tool for alleviating anxiety and pain in patients undergoing medical procedures. The mind is a powerful healing tool. Imagery (visualization) has harnessed the power of the mind through various therapies for centuries.

Creating images in your mind can reduce pain and other symptoms tied to your condition. The more specific the visualization, the more helpful it will likely be. People are taught to imagine sights, sounds, smells, tastes, or other sensations to create a kind of daydream that "removes" them from or gives them control over their present circumstances. Imagery usually involves a program with specific aims and goals. You are guided to visualize your goals and work toward them.

## How to?

By visualizing our goals and aspirations, we can manifest them into reality and stay motivated and focused on our path to success. Guided visualization exercises can help patients visualize positive outcomes and overcome negative thoughts and feelings. Visualize a positive result as if it has already been achieved. For example, if you are anxious about a job interview, visualize yourself completing the interview and getting the job.

In the context of Nursing, teach patient to use visualization to imagine themselves achieving their goals or overcoming obstacles. Encourage patients to practice visualization regularly and use it as a source of motivation and inspiration. By visualizing the desired outcome and holding positive intentions, nurses can amplify the energy around them and create a healing environment for themselves and their patients. Additionally, nurses can encourage patients to use prayer as a complementary therapy and provide resources for spiritual guidance and support.

## Visualization in Healthcare & Nursing

New Thought principles have also been integrated into nursing education and leadership frameworks. Specifically, the tenets of positive thinking and the law of attraction have been employed to assist nurses in overcoming challenges and achieving professional objectives. Research indicates that nurses who engage in positive self-talk and visualization techniques report higher levels of job satisfaction and are less prone to burnout (Decker & Borgen, 2002).

Two case studies highlight the potential benefits of incorporating New Thought principles into nursing practice. In one study, nurses received training using positive affirmations and visualization techniques aimed at reducing stress and enhancing job satisfaction. Post-training evaluations revealed that the nurses experienced lower stress levels and increased job satisfaction (Hernandez, 2009).

In another study, patients undergoing chemotherapy were taught visualization techniques to manage anxiety and pain. Following the visualization sessions, patients reported significant reductions in both anxiety and pain (Richardson & Smith, 1991).

<u>Two imagery techniques</u> are widely used today:

**Palming.** This involves visualizing color. You place your palms over your eyes and picture the color you think of with stress, usually red. Then, you change the color to a more relaxing color, such as blue. It is thought that changing colors in the mind helps you relax.

**Guided imagery.** This involves thinking of a particular goal to help cope with health problems. Guided imagery is most often used as a relaxation technique. It consists in sitting or lying quietly and imagining yourself in a favorite peaceful setting, such as a beach, meadow, or forest. Imagery could be guided by direct suggestions from a qualified imagery practitioner. Another example is when a person with cancer imagines Pac-Man (from the old Pac-Man video game) gobbling up bad cancer cells.

Studies have shown that imagery can help the mind and body relax. It can also help:

- Manage anxiety, stress, and depression
- Help reduce pain
- Lower blood pressure
- Lessen nausea
- Give you a better sense of control and well-being

Correspondingly, it is justified to include the effects of techniques like Mindfulness in healthcare. The high relapse rates following substance misuse treatment emphasize the urgent need for more effective therapies. A systematic review assessed the methodological characteristics and key outcomes of studies on mindfulness treatments for substance misuse published up to 2015. It also included the first meta-analysis of randomized controlled trials focused on mindfulness interventions for substance misuse. (Li, W., Howard et al., 2017).

Comprehensive searches in PubMed, PsycINFO, and Web of Science identified 42 relevant studies. The meta-analysis revealed that mindfulness treatments had small-to-large positive effects in reducing both the frequency and severity of substance misuse, the intensity of cravings for psychoactive substances, and the severity of stress. Additionally, mindfulness treatments proved more effective in promoting post-treatment abstinence from cigarette smoking when compared to other therapeutic approaches.

Another example is the case of Dr. Carl Simonton, who developed a mind-body approach to cancer treatment that included visualization, positive affirmations, and meditation. He reported many instances of patients who had complete remissions of their cancer after adopting his approach. There are also numerous anecdotal reports of individuals who have experienced spontaneous remissions of cancer after adopting a positive mindset, engaging in meditation and visualization, and making lifestyle changes that prioritize self-care and self-love.

Dr. Carl Simonton's book "Getting Well Again" describes the case of a woman with ovarian cancer who underwent a program of visualization and imagery, along with other complementary therapies. She experienced a complete remission and was cancer-free for over five years.

Overall, mindfulness-based interventions show promise as an effective treatment for substance misuse. However, further research is necessary to understand how these interventions work and to explore their effectiveness across diverse treatment environments. In Nursing, we must teach patients to practice mindfulness meditation, including deep breathing, body scanning, and visualization. Encourage the patient to practice for a few minutes daily and gradually increase the duration.

In summary, applying New Thought principles in nursing practice offers considerable potential. Positive thinking, visualization, and the mind-body connection can improve patients' outcomes, reduced stress, and enhanced job satisfaction among nurses.

## The Relationship Between the Mind, Body and Consciousness

Joe Dispenza is a world-renowned authority on the power of the mind-body connection. He started by traveling the world and interviewing people who had experienced what he calls "spontaneous remission" — a miraculous healing of terminal medical conditions.

Dr. Joe Dispenza's journey of becoming the world-renowned expert he is today began when he was seriously injured during a triathlon. He was on his bike while turning at an intersection when a four-wheel-drive Bronco going 55 mph hit him from behind. He landed hard on his back and broke six of the vertebrae in his spine. That injury should have been crippling. With so much damage to his spinal cord, Dr. Joe was lucky to be alive. He got four different opinions on how he should treat his injuries, and all four surgeons recommended a complicated operation called Harrington rod surgery, which would have required him to have steel rods surgically implanted in his back to realign his spinal cord. However, Dr. Joe did not want the surgery. He knew that having the surgery would mean committing to a life of being handicapped, and he just was not ready to give up yet. So, what did he do?

He practiced meditation and visualization. He imagined his spine repairing itself. Believe it or not, it worked! Dr. Joe's spine fully healed from his injuries, and just three months later, he was back on his feet and in training. All the doctors and surgeons he talked to told him he would be in a full-body cast for a year and disabled for life, but through the power of meditation, Dr. Joe used his mind to heal his body.

In his own words, Dr. Joe Dispenza shares:

"I thought I might as well take a chance here ... I think this voice kept coming up in my head, saying [that] the power that made the body heals the body. And I thought, '... This power is intelligence. Furthermore, intelligence is consciousness. Consciousness is awareness. Awareness is paying attention. It must be paying attention to me.' ... And I said, 'I am not going to let any thought slip by my awareness that I do not want to experience.' ... And so ... I just started reconstructing my spine in my mind, vertebrae by vertebrae."

Expert insights suggest that Dispenza's work is grounded in scientific research and offers practical personal growth and transformation tools. However, some experts caution against overgeneralizing the findings of neuroscience and quantum physics and encourage critical thinking and skepticism in interpreting these fields' concepts. Furthermore, while Dispenza's work emphasizes the role of individual agency and mindset in achieving goals and healing, experts caution against ignoring the systemic and social factors that may impact individuals' lives and opportunities.

Overall, the theory proposed in this chat and Dispenza's work focuses on the mind-body connection and the role of positive thinking and emotions in achieving health and well-being. By integrating insights from multiple fields, including nursing, neuroscience, and quantum physics, practitioners can adapt to a more polished and holistic approach to patient care.

## Intention, Visualization, and the New Thought Authors

Visualization is a powerful tool used by various renowned personalities. One such figure is Tim Ferriss, who uses Visualization to achieve his goals. Timothy Ferriss is an American entrepreneur, investor, author, podcaster, and lifestyle guru. He is known for his 4-Hour self-help book series—including the 4-Hour Work Week, the 4-Hour Body, and the 4-Hour Chef—which focused on lifestyle optimizations, but he has since reconsidered this approach. He recommends creating a vision board or visualization practice to help clarify goals and increase motivation.

The Master Key System is a self-help guide for personal growth and success based on the principles of the law of attraction and creative visualization by Charles F. Haanel. It was initially published as a 24-week correspondence course in 1912 and then in book form in 1916. The ideas it describes and explains come mostly from New Thought philosophy. It was one of the primary sources of inspiration for Rhonda Byrne's film and book The Secret (2006). Byrne promotes that visualizing one's desires can help manifest them into reality. A mindfulness-based approach could also incorporate visualization techniques, such as guided imagery, to help individuals focus on positive outcomes and reduce stress.

Prentice Mulford's book Thoughts Are Things will help you use the power of your thoughts to improve your life and to bring yourself the peace of mind you have always wished for. You will be able to learn how to think in a way that will help you succeed and make you happier in every aspect of your life. This book holds the Secret to the Law of Attraction! It also aligns with nursing, where it is essential to acknowledge the power of positive thinking and its impact on health and wellness. A mindful approach to self-healing and wellness nursing theory involves cultivating positive attitudes and emotions, such as gratitude, love, and compassion, and using visualization and positive affirmations to create a healthy mindset.

In his book The Power of Your Unconscious Mind, Joseph Murphy highlights the importance of visualization and positive affirmations in harnessing the power of the unconscious mind.

Murphy's work on the power of the unconscious mind provides valuable insights into how our thoughts and beliefs can shape our health and well-being. It offers practical strategies for harnessing the power of the mind to promote healing and positive change. These insights are highly relevant to the nursing theory being developed in this chat, which emphasizes the importance of mind-body approaches to healthcare and the role of positive thinking and mindfulness in promoting health and wellness.

These authors' work emphasizes the power of positive thinking, visualization, and the law of attraction and provide practical techniques for readers to use in order to manifest their desires and improve their lives. The new thought authors referenced in the book, such as Wallace Wattles, Napoleon Hill, and William Walker Atkinson, share common themes related to the power of positive thinking, visualization, and the law of attraction. These themes emphasize the role of positive emotions, mindfulness, and self-care in promoting healing and wellness.

## The Power of Manifestation

Neville Goddard, a Bajan writer, speaker, and mystic, taught various self-help methods to test his claim that the human imagination is omniscient and, therefore, God. His teachings continue to inspire countless individuals seeking to harness the power of their minds to create their desired realities. Neville's journey began with a deep curiosity about the nature of reality and the mind's potential. He explored various spiritual and metaphysical traditions, ultimately developing his unique approach to manifestation. Unlike many of his contemporaries, Neville emphasized the practical application of spiritual principles in everyday life. His teachings are grounded in the belief that everyone possesses the innate ability to shape their reality through the power of imagination and assumption.

At the center of Neville Goddard's philosophy lies the principle that imagination creates reality. He posited that by vividly envisioning one's desires as already fulfilled, individuals can bring them into existence. The following are some of his fundamental teachings:

**The Law of Assumption**

The law of assumption is one of Neville's most foundational concepts. According to this principle, whatever one assumes to be true ultimately becomes one's reality. By assuming the emotional state of having one's desires fulfilled, individuals initiate the processes necessary for those desires to materialize. This perspective challenges traditional views of cause and effect, suggesting that internal states of mind directly shape external circumstances.

Neville likened assumptions to seeds planted in the unconscious mind, which, when nurtured through persistence, eventually manifest in one's life. This method calls for a shift from superficial wishful thinking to a profound emotional conviction that one's desires have already been realized. By aligning both thought and emotion with the desired outcome, individuals become the creators of their reality.

*Neville Goddard's Law of Assumption posits that reality is shaped by one's internal beliefs and assumptions. According to this principle, the subconscious mind plays a crucial role in manifesting experiences, as it accepts whatever is impressed upon it as accurate and externalizes it into reality. This concept closely aligns with the idea of the subconscious mind as a portal to the divine matrix, where thoughts, emotions, and deeply held assumptions influence the fundamental structure of existence.*

*Goddard emphasized that assumption creates reality, suggesting that when an individual consistently holds a belief or mental state, it is absorbed by the subconscious mind and reflected in the external world. This aligns with the notion that the subconscious mind serves as the conduit to the divine matrix, where mental impressions interact with the deeper energetic framework of reality.*

*Scientific and philosophical perspectives, including quantum mechanics and the unified field theory, suggest that the observer influences the material world. This mirrors Goddard's assertion that individuals, through their assumptions and states of mind shape their lived experiences.*

*Mental clarity and focus are essential for the Law of Assumption to be effective. When the mind is free from distractions, such as during meditation, prayer, or deep contemplation, it becomes more receptive to internalized assumptions. This reflects the principle that when the mind is at peace and without external stimulus, the connection to the divine matrix is clearer.*

*Practices such as visualization and feeling the wish fulfilled—key techniques in Goddard's teachings—resonate with the idea that the subconscious mind, when properly directed, can influence the fundamental structure of reality. This supports the notion that aligning thought, emotion, and belief with a desired state creates a vibrational match with the divine matrix, leading to manifestation.*

*The Law of Assumption and the subconscious mind's connection to the divine matrix share a foundational premise: consciousness shapes reality. By impressing assumptions, intentions, and focused thoughts onto the subconscious, individuals can align with the deeper energetic field that governs existence. This perspective bridges the gap between metaphysical traditions, modern psychology, and quantum consciousness, offering a profound insight into the role of the mind and belief in manifesting personal and collective realities.*

## The Power of Imagination

For Neville, imagination was not merely a mental exercise but a creative force that shapes one's life. He emphasized the significance of using imagination to visualize goals vividly. Through the practice of sensory-rich mental imagery, individuals impress their unconscious mind with the reality of their aspirations. This technique dissolves the gap between one's present state and the desired future.

Neville frequently used the analogy of a film director to illustrate the role of imagination. Just as a director envisions every scene in intricate detail before filming, individuals must construct detailed mental images of their desired outcomes. This process extends beyond visualization; it necessitates complete immersion in the imagined experience, engaging all senses and emotions to enhance its impact on reality.

Goddard's teachings encourage individuals to visualize and feel their desired outcomes, which can be applied to nursing by encouraging patients to participate actively in their own healing process. In nursing practice, visualization techniques can help patients reduce stress and anxiety and increase their sense of control over their health outcomes. By promoting positive visualization and mindfulness techniques, patients can better manage their symptoms and improve their overall quality of life.

## How to Manifest in Five Steps

Here is a teaching guide for teaching patients the concept of manifesting their desired outcomes through visualization and positive thinking using the teachings of Neville Goddard:

**Step 1: Introduce the concept of visualization and positive thinking**

Explain to the patient that their thoughts and emotions can significantly impact their overall health and well-being. Discuss the concept of visualization and how it can help to manifest desired outcomes. Explain that positive thinking can help reduce stress, anxiety, and negative thought patterns, improving mental and physical health.

**Step 2: Explain the process of visualization and manifestation**

Discuss the importance of setting clear goals and intentions. Explain that visualization involves imagining and feeling the desired outcome as if it has already happened. Encourage the patient to create a mental picture of their desired outcome and focus on its positive emotions. Explain that the more the patient can feel the feelings associated with their desired outcome, the more likely it is to manifest.

**Step 3: Provide examples of visualization and manifestation**

Provide real-life examples of how visualization and manifestation have helped other patients to achieve their desired outcomes. Explain how positive thinking and visualization can improve physical health, such as reducing pain or improving the immune system. Encourage the patient to share their personal experiences with positive thinking and manifestation.

**Step 4: Provide practical strategies for visualization and manifestation**

Encourage the patient to set aside time daily for visualization and positive thinking. Suggest that the patient create a vision board or visualization journal to help them stay focused on their desired outcomes. Teach the patient relaxation techniques such as deep breathing and meditation to help them get into a relaxed state for visualization.

**Step 5: Encourage the patient to track their progress and celebrate their successes**

Encourage the patient to track their progress and celebrate their successes. Discuss any setbacks or challenges that may arise and encourage the patient to stay focused on their goals. Remind the patient that positive thinking and visualization are lifelong practices that require dedication and consistency.

The Law of Attraction or Manifestation is not a new concept. It has been recognized and practiced by many cultures throughout history. For example, the ancient Egyptians believed in the power of visualization and used it to create their reality. Recently, it was popularized by authors such as Napoleon Hill and Dale Carnegie. Napoleon Hill is the author of the classic book "Think and Grow Rich," which emphasizes the importance of positive thinking and visualization in achieving success. He believed individuals could manifest their desired outcomes by focusing on positive thoughts and beliefs.

# Jean Watson's Carative Principles and the Power of Intention & Visualization

*In Nursing, positive visualization can promote positive thinking and reduce anxiety or stress. Nurses can use positive visualization in several ways, such as imagining a successful patient outcome or a positive interaction with a colleague. For example, a nurse can use positive visualization before a challenging patient interaction. The nurse can promote a positive attitude and reduce stress by imagining a positive outcome, such as the patient responding well to treatment or expressing gratitude for the care received.*

*Jean Watson's Theory of Human Caring aligns deeply with the idea that consciousness plays a vital role in healing. Her carative factors emphasize the mind-body connection, the power of intention, and the role of energy and presence in fostering well-being. This perspective resonates with research in quantum consciousness, the subconscious mind, and holistic healing, all of which suggest that human thought, emotion, and belief influence health and reality.*

*Watson's approach highlights that love, compassion, and intentional presence are not just psychological comforts but active healing forces. This connects with the idea that the subconscious mind acts as a portal to the divine matrix, where belief systems, emotions, and focused thought influence physical and emotional health.*

*Studies in psychoneuroimmunology suggest that positive emotional states, such as those cultivated through caring interactions, reduce stress hormones and enhance immune function. This aligns with Watson's principle of creating a healing environment by addressing physical needs and emotional, mental, and spiritual well-being.*

*Watson's emphasis on being authentically present and engaging in transpersonal caring mirrors practices found in meditation, prayer, and energy healing modalities. The idea that focused intention and loving-kindness can enhance healing aligns with:*

*The placebo effect demonstrates that belief and expectation influence biological outcomes. Quantum consciousness theories suggest that observation and intention interact with the fabric of reality. The Law of Assumption (Neville Goddard) reinforces that deeply held beliefs shape experiences.*

*One of Watson's foundational beliefs is that love is the core of healing. This directly parallels the idea that love, consciousness, and the divine matrix are interconnected. If consciousness is the fundamental creative force of reality, then love—its most potent and cohesive expression—is the essence of healing.*

*Jean Watson's carative principles are more than a humanistic nursing model; they provide a scientific and spiritual framework that aligns with the deeper workings of consciousness, the subconscious mind, and the energetic nature of reality. Overall, it is essential to emphasize that positive thinking and visualization are tools that patients can use to take an active role in their own healthcare and improve their overall well-being. By teaching patients these concepts and providing practical strategies for implementation, nurses can empower patients to take control of their health and achieve their desired outcomes.*

One significant takeaway from this exploration is the idea that the mind and body are interconnected. The mind-body connection has been well-documented in numerous studies, and the evidence affirms that our thoughts and emotions can have a significant impact on our physical health (Lipton, 2015; Segerstrom & Miller, 2004). Additionally, positive thought and intention have been linked to improved patient outcomes, including pain management, decreased anxiety, and shorter hospital stays (Lengacher et al., 2018; Sturgeon et al., 2016; Vranceanu et al., 2014).

*Healing is not merely a physical process but a convergence of belief, intention, love, and energy, reinforcing that the mind is a powerful tool in shaping health and well-being.* Nurses who practice self-care and maintain a balanced energy state are better equipped to provide compassionate and effective care. This approach aligns with the idea that the nurse's energy and intentions can influence the healing process, both for themselves and for their patients. By fostering their well-being, nurses can enhance their ability to connect with patients on a deeper level and support their healing journey.

Furthermore, nurses can encourage patients to adopt healthy lifestyle behaviors, including a nutritious diet, regular exercise, and stress management techniques. By educating patients on the mind-body connection and the importance of positive thought and intention, nurses can empower patients to take an active role in their health and wellness.

The New Nursing recognizes that every person is a unique and interconnected energy system, and that health is achieved through the balance and harmonization of this energy. It also acknowledges the power of intention and positive emotions in promoting healing and wellness. By applying the New Nursing Theory, nurses can use intention, prayer, meditation, and visualization techniques to focus their intention on promoting healing and wellness. They can create a healing environment that supports the patient's physical, emotional, and spiritual needs. They can also incorporate other complementary and alternative therapies, such as acupuncture and energy healing, to support the balance and harmony of the patient's energy system.

The Universal Connectivity Theory can be applied in various healthcare settings, including acute care, long-term care, and community health. Healthcare providers can utilize mindfulness, visualization, and positive affirmations to facilitate the connection of patients to the universal force for healing and wellness. Collaborative care can be achieved through open communication and shared decision-making between healthcare providers and patients.

Patients can be taught to incorporate mindfulness, visualization, and positive affirmations into their daily lives to facilitate the connection to the universal force. Patient education efforts can focus on the importance of being present and aware of one's thoughts and emotions, the power of visualization and positive affirmations, and the benefits of collaborative care.

As a practical application of the theory, practitioners would utilize techniques such as visualization, meditation, and intention setting to direct energy toward positive outcomes. These techniques have significantly impacted health outcomes, including pain reduction, improved immune function, and increased well-being. In addition, using sound and vibrational therapies, such as music, chanting, and toning, can also profoundly affect the energy field, promoting healing and reducing negative energy.

As healthcare professionals, we can incorporate these principles into our practice. By acknowledging the interconnectedness of all things and the power of thoughts, emotions, and intentions, healthcare professionals can support patients in achieving optimal health and well-being.

## References

**"The Doctrine of Vibration"** by Mark S. G. Dyczkowski provides an excellent explanation of Spanda and its role in Shaiva Tantra.

**"The Triadic Heart of Shiva"** by Paul E. Muller-Ortega explores Abhinavagupta's teachings on the nature of divine consciousness.

Gregg Bradon, The Divine Matrix: Bridging Time, Space, Miracles, and Belief, 2007.

Gregg Braden – The Spontaneous Healing Of Belief: Shattering The Paradigm Of False Limits

Britannica, The Editors of Encyclopaedia. "intention". *Encyclopedia Britannica*, 29 Feb. 2012, https://www.britannica.com/topic/intention-logic. Accessed 29 September 2024.

MCTAGGART, L. (2007). The intention experiment: Using your thoughts to change your life and the world. New York: Simon & Schuster.

Emoto, M. (2004). The Hidden Messages in Water. Atria Books.

Li, W., Howard, M. O., Garland, E. L., McGovern, P., & Lazar, M. (2017). Mindfulness treatment for substance misuse: A systematic review and meta-analysis. Journal of Substance Abuse Treatment, 75, 62-96. https://doi.org/10.1016/j.jsat.2017.01.008

Dr. Joe Dispenza - The Relationship Between the Mind, Body and Consciousness.

Simonton, C. O., Matthews-Simonton, S., & Creighton, J. L. (1978). Getting well again. Bantam.

Lipton, B. H. (2015). The biology of belief 10th-anniversary edition: Unleashing the power of consciousness, matter & miracles. Hay House, Inc.

Lengacher, C. A., Reich, R. R., Post-White, J., Moscoso, M. S., Shelton, M. M., Barta, M. K., ... & Goodman, M. (2018). Mindfulness-based stress reduction (MBSR (BC)) in breast cancer survivors: symptom outcomes and biomarkers. Cancer Nursing, 41(4), 271-278.

# Chapter 5: THE BUTTERFLY EFFECT

Small Acts, Monumental Shifts in Healing

## Overview

What if the most powerful medicine in healing was felt, not measured; offered, not prescribed? When, in the chaos of a hospital ward, amidst beeping machines and sterile walls, a nurse offers a moment of deep presence, a soft gaze, a held hand, and a whisper of hope, it may seem trivial. But, like the butterfly's wings, that small gesture rides on waves of energy, intention, and love—rippling through the patient's body. It calms their nervous system, lighting up neural pathways, and perhaps even nudging the universe to co-conspire and accelerate the healing process.

This is the Butterfly Effect. It fits elegantly into *Powers of Love and Mind in Healing*, especially when tied to *quantum entanglement, the Law of Attraction*, and *nursing practice*. This chapter explores how subtle, loving acts in caregiving, especially in nursing, can create powerful ripples in a patient's healing journey. Using the lens of the Butterfly Effect, quantum entanglement, and the law of attraction, we will explore how the most minor shift in mindset, energy, and action can lead to profound physiological and emotional outcomes.

The Theory of Chaos, which delves into the science of surprises and focuses on the nonlinear and the inherently unpredictable, has practical applications in healthcare. It emphasizes the importance of anticipating the unexpected. While traditional sciences often address phenomena that are considered predictable, such as gravity, electricity, or chemical reactions, Chaos Theory examines nonlinear systems that are intrinsically difficult to forecast or control—examples include turbulence, weather patterns, stock market fluctuations, and the dynamics of brain states.

These phenomena are frequently described using fractal mathematics, which captures the boundless complexity found in nature. Numerous natural structures, including landscapes, clouds, trees, organs, and river systems, display fractal characteristics. Many systems in which we exist exhibit intricate, chaotic behavior. Recognizing these systems' chaotic and fractal nature can provide us with a deeper understanding, enhanced control, and greater wisdom.

For instance, by comprehending the intricate and chaotic dynamics of the atmosphere, a balloon pilot can strategically navigate a balloon toward a specific destination. Similarly, understanding the interconnected nature of ecological, social, and economic systems can help us avoid actions that might otherwise have adverse effects on our long-term well-being.

*"It used to be thought that the events that changed the world were things like big bombs, maniac politicians, huge earthquakes, or vast population movements, but it has now been realized that this is a very old-fashioned view held by people totally out of touch with modern thought. The things that really change the world, according to Chaos theory, are the tiny things. A butterfly flaps its wings in the Amazonian jungle, and subsequently, a storm ravages half of Europe.* – from Good Omens by Neil Gaiman and Terry Practchett[xiv]

The world's vast and intricate nature often leads us to believe that our small decisions and actions have little influence on broader outcomes. However, closer reflection on the minute details of our lives reveals how seemingly trivial events can serve as catalysts for major changes. For instance, a chance encounter at a coffee shop might lead to a conversation with someone who works at your dream company, eventually resulting in a job interview. A slight alteration in circumstances—choosing a different coffee shop or arriving a few minutes later—could have entirely changed the trajectory of that encounter and, consequently, your career. This phenomenon, where minor actions can trigger substantial outcomes, is known as the butterfly effect.

The butterfly effect is grounded in the principle that the world is profoundly interconnected, wherein a small event can impact a much larger, complex system. Its name derives from an allegory in chaos theory, suggesting that the flap of a butterfly's wings might, under certain conditions, set off a typhoon elsewhere. The uncertainty lies in whether or not these small actions will lead to such chaotic outcomes, as predicting their ultimate influence on complex systems is exceedingly challenging.

## What is the Butterfly Effect?

Rooted in Chaos Theory, the Butterfly Effect illustrates how a minor perturbation in one part of a system can induce substantial and non-linear outcomes elsewhere.

This concept was first introduced by mathematician and meteorologist Edward Norton Lorenz in the early 1960s; however, ideas relating to the theory predate Lorenz's identification of the effect within a scientific context. Lorenz searched for ways to predict the weather accurately and found that mathematical linear models did not provide accurate predictions. Just as it would be almost impossible to predict that you would land your dream job by deciding to get coffee, Lorenz found that initial weather conditions were insufficient indicators of future weather conditions.

In 1963, Lorenz published a paper with these ideas titled *Deterministic Nonperiodic Flow*. In this paper, he essentially argued that weather predictions were inaccurate not only because knowing the precise starting conditions was impossible but also because a tiny degree of change throws off the results. He stressed that it didn't necessarily change the course of events, but that it could, and that there was essentially no way of knowing what caused changes in weather. Lorenz, therefore, advocated for deterministic chaos models that account for the exponential growth of errors.

The famous metaphor of a butterfly flapping its wings in one region of the world, resulting in a tornado forming in another week's later, suggested that even seemingly insignificant actions, such as a butterfly's wing movement in New Mexico, could eventually contribute to a hurricane in China. Though the time span may be extensive, the causal relationship is theoretically valid.

In more precise terms, small variations in initial conditions can lead to significant divergences in outcomes. This principle is continuously manifested in our lives. The long-term impacts of educating millions of children about concepts like chaos theory and fractals remain unpredictable yet potentially profound.

## The Butterfly Flap in the Healing Space

In 1961, meteorologist Edward Lorenz stumbled upon a phenomenon that would change how we view cause and effect: a small alteration in initial conditions, like the flap of a butterfly's wings, could set off a tornado weeks later. Known as the Butterfly Effect, this concept from chaos theory reveals that in sensitive systems, minor changes can lead to monumental outcomes.

The human body, psyche, and energy field are deeply sensitive systems. In a hospital room, where stress, fear, and uncertainty swirl, what happens when a nurse enters with presence, love, and calm intention? Is it just a moment of kindness—or the first flap of healing wings?

## Scientific Bridges: Chaos, Energy, and Entanglement

Healthcare often focuses on what is measurable, but quantum science teaches us that the most impactful phenomena may be invisible. In quantum entanglement, particles that interact once remain connected, no matter how far apart they move. A shift in one immediately affects the other. Undoubtedly, human beings, especially those in close physical or emotional proximity, are energetically entangled.

Nurses are entangled with their patients—not just physically, but emotionally, neurologically, and energetically. The field of Heart-Brain Coherence, explored by organizations like the HeartMath Institute, shows how heart-based emotions like love and gratitude regulate the nervous system and create a healing biofield. Presence becomes medicine.

Love is not merely a feeling—it is a frequency. Intentional thoughts, loving emotions, and silent prayers, all contribute to an unseen but potent energy field. The Law of Attraction proposes that like attracts like. In the context of healing, a nurse's conscious projection of love, hope, and wholeness can align the patient's energy field toward recovery.

Dr. Wayne Dyer called intention the starting point of every miracle. In a healing space, intention becomes the silent architect of outcomes. When paired with love, it becomes a force of nature.

Nurses operate at the frontlines of energy exchange. In every patient interaction, they offer more than medication—they offer presence. Their touch, their tone, and even their internal emotional state creates a ripple in the patient's field. Consider the concept of Energetic Nurseship: the practice of becoming aware of one's energy, intention, and emotional presence as tools of healing. The nurse becomes the butterfly, their smallest gesture the flap that might turn the tide of recovery.

## Where the Butterfly Danced – Some Micro and Macro Instances

*The Silent Prayer*: A nurse in the ICU begins to offer a silent blessing before tending to each unconscious patient. Over time, her patients showed improved stabilization.

*The Presence Shift*: After learning mindfulness, a nurse begins grounding herself before each interaction. Patients begin commenting on her calming presence. One terminal patient calls her "a beam of peace."

*The Ripple Beyond the Room*: A nurse notices a grieving mother and offers 15 minutes of listening. The mother later donates equipment to the hospital. Her act of grief became one of generosity—all because someone stopped to listen.

Each story is a living testament to the Butterfly Effect. One small act. One moment of love. One energetic shift. Monumental change.

Here are a few examples of Global events evident of the impact of the Butterfly Effect:

- **The Bombing of Nagasaki:** Cloud cover over the original target, Kuroko, led to Nagasaki being bombed instead. A simple weather change altered history.
- **Hitler's Art School Rejection:** Twice rejected from Art school at the Academy of Fine Arts in Vienna, Hitler's path changed from aspiring artist to dictator. Imagine if he had been accepted.
- **Archduke Franz Ferdinand's Assassination:** A wrong turn by his driver put him in the path of his assassin. This sparked World War I.

- **The Chornobyl Disaster:** Three workers prevented a second explosion that could have made half of Europe uninhabitable. Their actions limited the catastrophe.
- **The Cuban Missile Crisis:** One Russian officer, Vasili Arkhipov, vetoed launching a nuclear torpedo. He likely prevented World War III.

These examples show how small events could and can have enormous global-level consequences. The *Butterfly Effect* affirms that small changes can have far-reaching, sometimes unpredictable impacts—a concept that aligns well with the healthcare and nursing profession.

## The Butterfly Effect of Caring

The concept of the "Butterfly Effect of Caring"[xv] is a central metaphor, emphasizing the interconnectedness and ethical responsibilities in caregiving. This perspective highlights the moral imperative to respond compassionately to the vulnerability of others, with the visible suffering of another person invoking a call to empathetic action. One such research underscores that developing a compassionate self—characterized by sensitivity, non-judgment, and self-respect—directly contributes to the capacity for offering compassionate care to others.

Compassionate care is understood not merely as an action performed by the caregiver nor simply as a way of relating to or feeling for another person. Instead, it represents a mutual process of becoming and belonging, where the caregiver and the cared-for are actively engaged in a shared experience. In this process, the caregiver acknowledges and respects the mutual vulnerability and dignity of both themselves and those in their care.

Here is how the Butterfly Effect relates to nursing and healthcare:

1. **Patient Interactions and Outcomes:**

In nursing, even minor actions like a reassuring touch, a kind word, or a few extra minutes spent with a patient can significantly impact recovery. This idea parallels the Butterfly Effect: small gestures of care can set off a chain reaction, improving a patient's emotional state, fostering resilience, and ultimately contributing to faster recovery. A study in the *Journal of Clinical Nursing* emphasizes the importance of compassion in care, highlighting how small acts of kindness in nursing can reduce anxiety, improve patient satisfaction, and promote healing (Sinclair, S. et al., 2017).

2. **Systemic Changes and Health Outcomes:**

On a larger scale, minor policy changes or adjustments in care protocols within healthcare systems can significantly impact patient care outcomes. For example, introducing a new hand hygiene protocol might seem small. However, it has a profound impact, it can dramatically reduce infection rates, similar to how the Butterfly Effect affirms that minor changes can cause more significant shifts. The concept is well-articulated in *BMJ Quality & Safety*, where minor process improvements in healthcare practices have a cascading effect on patient outcomes (Dixon-Woods M. et al., 2011).

3. **Emotional and Psychological Effects:**

The impact of nursing extends beyond physical care to emotional and psychological well-being. A nurse's positive attitude and empathetic communication can create a ripple effect, improving patients' overall mood and engagement, which may positively influence their physiological healing processes. This aligns with the notion that small changes in emotional support can result in broader mental and physical health improvements. Research published in *Health Psychology* discusses the influence of emotional support on physical recovery, showing that even brief, positive interactions can lead to better health outcomes (Uchino, B. N., et al., 2006).

### *Becoming the Butterfly: Daily Practices for Nurses*

1. **Mindful Entry**: Pause before entering a room. Inhale with intention. Exhale with love.

2. **Heart-Centered Listening**: Listen not to reply, but to feel. Let your presence be a balm.

3. **Energetic Hygiene**: Clear your field daily—visualize light, breathe deeply, and shake off absorbed stress.

4. **Loving-Kindness Meditations**: Take 5 minutes before or after a shift to send love inward and outward.

These aren't just wellness tools—they are acts of sacred service. They are the butterfly wings.

We often seek healing in interventions, procedures, and technology. Yet, perhaps the truest medicine lies in the invisible: in presence, in love, in the conscious intention to hold another in wholeness. Like the butterfly's wings, the smallest act of love can change everything.

## 4. Holistic Care and the Ripple Effect:

The Butterfly Effect can also be seen in the holistic approach that many nurses adopt. Nurses create a more profound and enduring impact by addressing physical symptoms and the mental, emotional, and social aspects of a patient's life. This approach can transform a patient's experience, much like how a butterfly's wings can lead to significant changes in a distant place. *The Healing Environment: Without and Within* by Esther M. Sternberg touches on how holistic care practices, even if subtle, can have significant long-term effects on patient recovery (Sternberg, E. M., 2009).

## Conclusion

In this chapter, we dug deeper and found various references and examples to demonstrate how the Butterfly Effect metaphorically aligns with the field of Nursing and its practice. We examined how minor decisions in patient care or momentary interactions could have far-reaching consequences, shaping the course of healthcare outcomes in unpredictable yet profound ways.

"As far as the laws of mathematics refer to reality, they are not certain, and as far as they are certain, they do not refer to reality." - Albert Einstein.

Every thought we produce generates a vibration that resonates throughout the universe, with profound implications for both individual well-being and collective outcomes. Positive thoughts, characterized by love and compassion, can contribute to peace and happiness. At the same time, those driven by anger and greed may give rise to turmoil, even extending to natural disasters. This perspective is rooted in the principles of quantum mechanics, which, as described by Gregory J. Nicosia, Ph.D., offers a comprehensive framework for understanding the nature of reality. In his article, "Thought Energy: The Basis of a Quantum Leap in Psychotherapy," Nicosia emphasizes that quantum mechanics has revealed that every particle is accompanied by an "information wave," which guides its behavior.

From this standpoint, thought and intention are not merely abstract concepts but are integral to transforming energy from higher-dimensional, faster-than-light waveforms into the tangible, four-dimensional reality we experience. Nicosia conceptualizes thought energy fields as collections of related thoughts bound together by shared themes or experiences, functioning as cohesive units. He posits that thoughts emerge from energy, gradually slowing down until they solidify into matter, akin to a process frozen in time. In this view, the distinction between mind and matter becomes minimal—they represent different stages in manifesting our observable reality. This understanding offers profound insights into the role of intention in shaping outcomes, reinforcing the notion that even small shifts in thought can initiate significant changes in the context of healthcare and nursing practices.

The concept of the New Nursing Theory of Love relates to the Butterfly Effect through its emphasis on how small, seemingly insignificant actions, such as thoughts or intentions, can have far-reaching impacts on larger systems. Just as the Butterfly Effect affirms that the subtle flap of a butterfly's wings can set off a series of events leading to a much larger outcome, the idea of thought energy from quantum mechanics implies that even a single thought can initiate a chain of reactions that shape reality.

In both cases, the underlying theme is the interconnectedness of systems, where minute changes can lead to unpredictable and sometimes profound consequences. For example, in nursing and healthcare, the mindset and intentions of practitioners, whether grounded in compassion or negativity, can significantly influence patient outcomes, care dynamics, and even the broader healing environment. A compassionate thought or small act of kindness could ripple through patient interactions, fostering a culture of care that enhances recovery and well-being. Conversely, negative or dismissive attitudes could contribute to a less supportive environment, potentially impacting patient experiences and outcomes.

Thus, the principles of thought energy in quantum mechanics align with the Butterfly Effect's idea that small changes in initial conditions—a thought, action, or intention—can ultimately lead to larger, sometimes unpredictable shifts within a complex system. In the context of nursing and healthcare, this highlights the importance of mindful, compassionate engagement, as the cumulative impact of these small choices can transform the entire care ecosystem.

# Chapter 6: Case Studies in Mind-Body Healing

Over time, humanity's relationship with the natural environment has experienced a significant transformation, resulting in lifestyles that increasingly disconnect individuals from their surroundings. This disconnection has diminished the activation of ancient survival mechanisms, leading to a detachment from intrinsic physiological and mental resilience.

It is commonly understood that only a small portion of the brain is engaged in conscious thought. At the same time, the majority is dedicated to deeper processes governing a wide range of bodily functions. The ability to deliberately influence this more significant, subconscious part of the brain could offer unprecedented control over physiological processes, suggesting previously unattainable capabilities.

Through decades of personal exploration and pioneering scientific research, individuals like Wim Hof and Joe Dispenza have developed various effective methodologies to re-engage these foundational physiological processes, thereby facilitating the realization of human potential. In this chapter, we will examine Wim Hof and Joe Dispenza's case studies of mind-body healing.

## Wim Hof's Method

Wim Hof, commonly referred to as the "Iceman" (Muzik et al.), is a Dutch athlete known for his extraordinary resilience to extreme cold conditions. He has achieved world records related to cold endurance and pioneered a method that integrates controlled cold exposure, specialized breathing exercises, and meditation practices.

This chapter delves into the practical applications of Hof's method within nursing practice, emphasizing the influence of mental control over physiological responses. The Wim Hof Method is a powerful tool for reconnection to oneself, to others, and to the natural world.

Wim Hof's method is a unique wellness technique that harnesses the power of breathing exercises, cold exposure, and meditation to unlock the potential of the mind and body. This method is founded on the belief that exposure to cold temperatures can significantly enhance health and well-being.

Wim Hof's method is more of a practice than just a theory, based on solid evidence. It is rooted in the idea that the mind can exert control over the body. In a compelling experiment, Hof demonstrated his ability to regulate his body temperature while immersed in ice water, solely through the use of breathing exercises and mental focus.

Wim Hof's method consists of three key components:

- cold exposure
- breathing techniques
- meditation

Cold exposure involves exposing the body to freezing temperatures, which can range from cold showers to sitting in an ice bath. Breathing techniques involve a specific pattern of deep breathing and breath-holding. The meditation component consists in focusing the mind on positive thoughts and feelings.

**Cold Exposure:**

Cold exposure is a foundational component of the Wim Hof Method, and in recent years, cold therapy has gained significant popularity due to its association with various health benefits. Whole-body cryotherapy, in particular, is endorsed by numerous individuals, including professional athletes, bodybuilders, and public figures, who advocate for its benefits. This therapy involves briefly standing in a sealed chamber where extremely cold air circulates around the body.

Given that whole-body cryotherapy can be costly and is not widely accessible, the Wim Hof Method offers a practical and affordable alternative. By incorporating cold exposure practices such as cold showers, individuals can engage in cold therapy from the convenience of their homes and begin to experience its potential benefits.

## Breathing:

Breathing is among the most essential human functions. It initiates the crucial process of oxygen delivery that sustains all bodily functions continuously. Even minor adjustments to breathing patterns can exert significant and immediate effects on physiological processes.

This section highlights the practice of the Wim Hof Method breathing exercises and examines their effectiveness in managing stress, enhancing sleep, and supporting various aspects of health and well-being. Notably, these exercises are simple and time-efficient, requiring only a few minutes while offering lasting benefits.

*NOTE: Wim Hof Method breathing can affect motor control and, in rare cases, lead to loss of consciousness. Always sit or lie down when practicing the techniques. **Never practice in or near bodies of water**, while piloting a vehicle, or in any other situation where losing consciousness could cause harm to you or others.*

## Meditation:

The third pillar of the Wim Hof Method is meditation, which plays a crucial role in integrating the effects of breathwork and cold exposure. Meditation helps practitioners tap into the mind-body connection, fostering a sense of calm and balance. Wim Hof's guided meditation sessions often focus on mindfulness and gratitude, contributing to a holistic approach to well-being. Through meditation and conscious breathing, you can observe your thoughts, emotions, and impulses without identifying or acting on them. Willpower, self-control and commitment are very important parts of the Wim Hof Method because conscious breathing and cold therapy require patience and dedication. We believe you can train your brain to increase willpower and self-control. The exercises that are instructed by Wim all have a powerful effect on skills that relate to self-control. They improve your focus, reduce your stress levels and make you more self-aware.

## Health Benefits of the Wim Hof's Method

Several studies have explored the potential health benefits of Wim Hof's method. Here are some of the benefits of the Wim Hof Method:

- **Improved mental clarity**: The breathing exercises help increase oxygen levels in the body, which can promote a sense of calm and reduce stress.
- **Better immune function**: Cold exposure can help strengthen the immune system.
- **Increased energy**: Practitioners of the Wim Hof Method report increased energy and vitality.
- **Faster recovery**: The method can help with faster recovery from physical exertion.
- **Reduced inflammation**: The method can help reduce inflammation.

A study published in the Proceedings of the National Academy of Sciences found that Wim Hof's method can increase the body's resistance to stress and inflammation (Kox et al., 2014). Another study found that the method can improve immune function and reduce symptoms of depression (Meeusen et al., 2018). Additionally, a case study published in the Journal of Behavioral and Brain Science reported that the method can improve symptoms of chronic fatigue syndrome.

In another experiment, practitioners of the Wim Hof Method could control their sympathetic nervous system and immune response. After being trained in Wim's method, these participants were injected with an endotoxin (E. coli) and showed fewer symptoms, lower levels of pro-inflammatory mediators, and increased levels of plasma epinephrine—their immune systems were successfully battling the bacteria.

## Implications for Nursing Practice

Wim Hof's method has the potential to offer several benefits for nursing practice. It can be used as a tool to manage stress and improve immune function, which can be particularly beneficial for patients with chronic illnesses or those undergoing cancer treatment. Additionally, the method can help promote a sense of well-being and increase energy levels, which can benefit both patients and nurses.

Two case studies that demonstrate the potential benefits of Wim Hof's method are presented below:

### Case Study 1: Chronic Pain Management

A 40-year-old patient with chronic pain was referred to a nurse for pain management. The patient had been taking pain medication for several years, but the medication was no longer effective. The nurse recommended the patient to try Wim Hof's method, that reduced pain and inflammation. The patient was hesitant at first, but after practicing the method for several weeks, the patient reported a significant reduction in pain and was able to reduce their reliance on pain medication.

### Case Study 2: Anxiety Management

A 25-year-old patient with severe anxiety was admitted to the hospital for treatment. The patient had a history of anxiety and panic attacks and was prescribed medication to manage their symptoms. The nurse recommended that the patient try Wim Hof's method as an additional tool for managing their anxiety. The patient was initially skeptical, but after practicing the method for several days, the patient reported feeling more relaxed and less anxious. The patient was eventually able to reduce their reliance on medication and was discharged from the hospital with a plan to continue practicing the method.

The Wim Hof Method is a breathing technique developed by Dutch athlete Wim Hof that involves deep breathing exercises followed by breath retention. This technique is believed to increase energy levels and improve overall health and well-being.

## Wim Hof Method Teaching Plan:

This teaching plan can be adapted and customized to fit the specific needs and goals of the participants and setting. It is essential to ensure that the instructor is knowledgeable and experienced in the Wim Hof Method and to provide a safe and supportive learning environment for all participants.

### Introduction:

Introduce yourself as the instructor and provide a brief overview of the Wim Hof Method. Explain the purpose of the method, which is to improve overall health and well-being through breathing exercises, cold exposure, and meditation. Provide some background on Wim Hof and how he developed the method.

**Breathing Exercises:**

- Explain the breathing exercise in detail, including how to inhale deeply, exhale forcefully, and hold your breath.
- Demonstrate the breathing exercise to the group and have them follow along.
- Provide guidance and support to individuals who may be struggling with the exercise.
- Encourage participants to focus on their breath and try to clear their minds.

**Cold Exposure:**

- Explain the benefits of cold exposure, including improved circulation, reduced inflammation, and increased resilience to stress.
- Discuss the different methods of cold exposure, such as taking cold showers, immersing oneself in cold water, or standing in a cold room.
- Provide safety tips for cold exposure, including starting slowly and gradually increasing exposure time, monitoring body temperature and discomfort, and avoiding cold exposure when sick or pregnant.
- Encourage participants to start with shorter cold exposure sessions and gradually build up to longer periods.

**Meditation:**

- Explain the benefits of meditation, including reduced stress and anxiety, improved focus, and increased self-awareness.

- Discuss different meditation techniques, such as mindfulness meditation and loving-kindness meditation.
- Demonstrate a guided meditation and encourage participants to follow along.
- Provide guidance and support to individuals who may be struggling with meditation.

In the end, summarize the key points of the teaching plan and emphasize the importance of incorporating the Wim Hof Method into daily life. Provide additional resources and references for participants interested in learning more about the Wim Hof Method.

## Joe Dispenza's Work on Mind-Body Connection and Its Implications on Nursing

In the field of holistic health and personal transformation, Dr. Joe Dispenza is a prominent figure. As a neuroscientist, chiropractor, and international speaker, Dispenza has garnered a worldwide audience for his distinctive integration of scientific insights with spiritual practices. His approach emphasizes the potential of the mind to facilitate healing and personal transformation, based on the premise that by altering our thoughts, beliefs, and emotions, we can significantly impact physical health and enhance overall well-being.

Dr. Joe Dispenza conceptualizes the mind as to activate any neurological tissue within the brain or body, describing it as "the brain in action." He proposes that when consciousness engages neurological tissues, it generates what we perceive as the mind. Since each energy center in the body is associated with a nerve plexus, Dispenza affirms that each center may possess its own distinct "mind." While this idea may seem unconventional, he references common experiences—such as fantasizing or watching a movie—that trigger physiological responses in the reproductive area. During these experiences, the body releases specific chemicals and hormones from corresponding glands, priming the individual emotionally and energetically for sexual activity. In Dispenza's view, the "mind" associated with the reproductive area functions subconsciously through the autonomic nervous system, operating independently of conscious thought.

### The Core of Dr. Joe Dispenza's Philosophy

Dr. Joe Dispenza's works can also be related to the mindfulness-based approach to self-healing and wellness nursing theory.

At the heart of Dr. Dispenza's work is the belief that the mind has the power to heal the body. He teaches that by changing our thoughts and emotions, we can rewire our brains and influence our biology in profound ways. His philosophy is rooted in the idea that we are not victims of our genetics or environment but rather creators of our reality. We can shift our internal state and create measurable changes in our physical health and emotional well-being through meditation, visualization, and mind-body practices.

His teachings are grounded in several key concepts:

- Neuroplasticity – The brain's ability to reorganize itself by forming new neural connections.
- Epigenetics – The study of how behavior and environment can cause changes in the way genes are expressed.
- Quantum Physics – The understanding that consciousness can influence reality at the subatomic level.
- The Power of the Present Moment – The notion that healing occurs when we focus our attention on the present moment, free from past conditioning and future anxieties.

**Mind-body connection:**

Dr. Dispenza's work emphasizes the connection between the mind and body and how our thoughts and emotions can impact our physical health. This aligns with the concept of the carative factors in nursing theory, which emphasizes the importance of treating the whole person, not just the physical symptoms.

**Meditation and mindfulness:**

Dr. Dispenza is a proponent of meditation and mindfulness practices, which have been shown to have numerous health benefits, including reducing stress and improving mental and emotional well-being. These practices align with the concept of mindfulness-based approaches to healing and wellness and suggest that mindfulness-based therapy is a promising intervention for treating anxiety and mood problems in clinical populations (Hofmann, S. G., et al.).

Consciousness can be understood as comprising two primary, complementary dimensions: awareness of the sensory environment and awareness of action. Yoga Nidra, a meditative practice within the meditation tradition, allows for a subjective dissociation of these aspects, wherein the mind withdraws from the impulse to act. This state does not involve shifts in emotional states or willpower; instead, the meditator assumes the role of a neutral observer, experiencing a release of conscious control over actions alongside an intensification of sensory perception or imagination. Research findings indicate that meditation—whether within the Yoga Nidra framework or outside it—is characterized by a "profound willingness to relinquish personal goals and concerns, coupled with an intense absorption of attention" toward sensory experience. (Kjaer, T. W., et al.)

**Self-Awareness and Personal Transformation:** Dr. Dispenza's work emphasizes the importance of self-awareness and personal transformation in achieving optimal health and well-being. This aligns with the carative factors in nursing theory, which emphasize the importance of developing a caring relationship with patients and empowering them to take control of their own health and well-being.

Overall, the principles of mindfulness, self-awareness, and the mind-body connection that underlie Dr. Dispenza's work are consistent with the mindfulness-based approach to self-healing and wellness nursing theory.

## How Dr. Joe Dispenza's Approach Can Facilitate Healing

Dr. Joe Dispenza's approach offers a transformative perspective on healing, focusing on harnessing the mind's power to activate the body's inherent self-healing mechanisms rather than solely depending on external treatments. Here are several ways his work may support the healing process:

1. ***Reduces Stress and Anxiety*** – Through meditation and practices that align the heart and brain, Dispenza's methods help regulate stress hormones like cortisol, fostering a calm state for healing.
2. ***Enhances Physical Healing***—Numerous individuals practicing Dispenza's techniques report spontaneous remissions and health improvements. By shifting from states of fear or stress to those of love and gratitude, the body can more effectively channel energy toward healing processes.
3. ***Promotes Emotional Balance***—Dispenza's insights on emotional coherence encourage releasing negative emotional patterns, resulting in greater emotional resilience, inner peace, and stability.
4. ***Cultivates a Positive Mindset***—By rewiring neural pathways, individuals can replace limiting beliefs with empowering ones, facilitating transformations in health, relationships, career success, and overall quality of life.

In 2007, Wim Hof was examined by the well-known Feinstein Institute. The results showed that Wim Hof appeared to be able to influence his autonomic nervous system. According to various tests, the WHM has a number of health benefits. The Endotoxin experiment and the publication of this particular test in PNAS showed that Wim Hof and the test subjects who took part in the training sessions produced more stress hormones such as cortisol and adrenaline.

Stress hormones suppress inflammatory bodies in the bloodstream. For example, those suffering from an overactive immune system could benefit greatly from this. Furthermore, the brown fat tissue examination showed that Hof still had brown fat. This indicates that practicing the WHM has a favorable effect on maintaining brown fat levels. The following is a description of the effects of the WHM on various types of physical illnesses.

Dr. Joe Dispenza's work is more than just a healing method; it is a guide for personal transformation. By teaching us how to align our thoughts, emotions, and intentions, Dispenza empowers us to take control of our own health and well-being. His approach offers a powerful reminder that the body has an incredible ability to heal itself when the mind and heart are aligned in coherence. Whether you seek physical recovery, emotional balance, or spiritual growth, Dr. Joe Dispenza's teachings provide the tools to unlock your fullest healing potential.

These unique methodologies have proven to be successful in healthcare and the practice of Nursing as alternate modes of Healing for patients, further strengthening the basis of the New Nursing Theory of Mind and Love.

# References

Hofmann, S. G., Sawyer, A. T., Witt, A. A., & Oh, D. (2010). The effect of mindfulness-based therapy on anxiety and depression: A meta-analytic review. Journal of Consulting and Clinical Psychology, 78(2), 169-183. https://pubmed.ncbi.nlm.nih.gov/20350028/

Kox, M., van Eijk, L. T., Zwaag, J., van den Wildenberg, J., Sweep, F. C., van der Hoeven, J. G., & Pickkers, P. (2014). Voluntary activation of the sympathetic nervous system and attenuation of the innate immune response in humans. Proceedings of the National Academy of Sciences, 111(20), 7379-7384.

Meeusen, R., Watson, P., Hasegawa, H., Roelands, B., & Piacentini, M. F. (2018). Central fatigue: the serotonin hypothesis and beyond. Sports Medicine, 48(11), 2561-2579

Muzik, Otto & Reilly, Kaice & Diwadkar, Vaibhav. (2018). "Brain over body"–A study on the willful regulation of autonomic function during cold exposure. NeuroImage. 172. 10.1016/j.neuroimage.2018.01.067.

Kjaer, T. W., Bertelsen, C., Piccini, P., Brooks, D. J., & Alving, J. (2002). Increased dopamine tone during meditation-induced change of consciousness. Cognitive Brain Research, 13(2), 255-259. https://doi.org/10.1016/s0926-6410(01)00106-9

Dispenza, J. (2017). *Becoming Supernatural: How common people are doing the uncommon.* Carlsbad, CA: Hay House.

# Chapter 7: Emotions and Health

As we dive deeper into quantum physics and its connection to the universe, we uncover that everything around us operates as energy, frequency, and vibration. Our thoughts and emotions, integral components of this energetic spectrum, hold the power to influence our health and shape our reality. The energy we put out into the universe attracts similar energy back to us, and by aligning our thoughts, emotions, and actions with our goals, we can manifest our desires into reality.

This chapter discusses the influence of emotions on physical health outcomes. Emotions like happiness, resilience, and the avoidance of all sorts of negative emotions.

The American Psychological Association (APA) defines emotions as subjective mental reactions involving behavioral and physical responses. In short, emotions can affect the mind, actions, and body. Learning to recognize and cope with our emotions can help prevent negative mental and physical health-related consequences and improve our relationships and day-to-day life.

The idea that thoughts and emotions influence our reality is not new. Many spiritual traditions and ancient cultures have discussed this notion for centuries. The quantum nursing theory builds on this idea, recognizing that as energetic beings, our thoughts and emotions play a significant role in our physical, mental, and emotional health.

Persistent negative attitudes, along with feelings of helplessness and hopelessness, can lead to chronic stress. This prolonged stress disrupts hormonal equilibrium, depletes essential happiness-related neurotransmitters, and impairs immune function. Additionally, chronic stress has been linked to a reduction in lifespan. Scientific research indicates that stress accelerates the shortening of telomeres, the protective "end caps" of DNA strands, thereby hastening the aging process.

Poorly managed or repressed anger (hostility) is also related to a slew of health conditions, such as hypertension (high blood pressure), <u>cardiovascular disease</u>, <u>digestive disorders</u>, and infection.

Recent studies have also shown that our thoughts and emotions directly impact our physiology. Dr. Candace Pert, a neuroscientist and pharmacologist, has shown that emotions are not just abstract feelings but have a physical basis in our bodies. According to her research, emotions are molecules circulating throughout the body and can influence the immune system, nervous system, and other physiological processes.

The quantum nursing theory recognizes the power of our thoughts and emotions and their ability to influence our health. By understanding and harnessing this power, we can promote healing and well-being.

## Human Emotions and the Human Body

Each emotion you feel is designed to provoke a specific reaction in your body through hard-wired sensations and impulses. Many people believe these hard-wired responses are there to ensure your survival. For instance, feeling angry may trigger a <u>fight response</u>, while fear may cause you to flee (or have a "flight" response).[xvi]

Nevertheless, these impulses also can cause you to do or say things you wish you did not—especially, if you cannot recognize why you are feeling the way you do. Even when you know your emotions or feelings, your emotions can still exert a force on your body for a specific behavior. But, you can find ways to not act on every impulse and choose to respond in a different way.[5]

When considering how emotions affect mental health, it is essential to first note that no emotion is genuinely "bad" or negative. Instead, negative emotions signal that something is wrong and needs to be addressed.[xvii]

That said, if you struggle to manage these negative emotions or attempt to ignore or repress them when they crop up, this could negatively affect your mental health. In fact, when negative emotions persist for a long period of time—like chronic sadness, anger, or fear—this can lead to <u>depression</u>, <u>anxiety</u>, and even <u>substance use</u>.[xviii]

## How Emotions Affect Your Physical Health

Researchers have found a link between positive emotions and physical health. People with a positive outlook on life tend to have better overall health, including <u>lower blood pressure</u> and <u>blood sugar levels</u> and a reduced risk for <u>heart disease</u>. However, researchers do not know if these positive emotions lead to better health or if having good health leads to positive emotions. Experts theorize it may be a combination of both factors.[10]

There is also some evidence that experiencing positive emotions can affect recovery when you are sick or injured. In one study, researchers noted that a positive outlook can influence how quickly you get well and even influence survival rates.[xix]

Meanwhile, negative emotions have been tied to long-term adverse health effects. People who have trouble managing their emotions effectively or live with <u>stress</u> may be more likely to experience chronic health conditions and increase their risk of early death.[xx]

Lisa Feldman Barrett, a psychologist and neuroscientist, has demonstrated in her research that emotions are constructions that our brains create to guide our actions and explain how we feel in a specific situation. They are also, she is careful to point out, as real as anything we see, hear, or taste. In *How Emotions Are Made*, she emphasizes the profound connection between emotions and physical health. She argues that emotions significantly influence health outcomes through their role in managing the body's physiological state, particularly via the concept of *body budgeting*.

**Key Points on Emotions and Health:**

1. **Body-Budgeting**

   Barrett introduces the idea of a "body's budget," where the brain allocates energy resources to maintain physical well-being. Emotions play a crucial role in this process by preparing the body for action or recovery. For example:

   - Stress and anxiety can drain the body's budget, leading to chronic inflammation, weakened immunity, or cardiovascular strain.
   - Positive emotions, like joy or contentment, can replenish the body-budget, promoting recovery and long-term health.

2. **Chronic Stress and Illness**

   Prolonged negative emotional states, such as chronic stress or fear, can disrupt the balance of the body-budget. This can lead to various health problems, including:

   - High blood pressure
   - Digestive issues

- Increased risk of heart disease
- Sleep disturbances

3. **Emotional Granularity and Health**

Barrett highlights the importance of *emotional granularity*—the ability to distinguish between different emotional states precisely. People with higher emotional granularity are better at managing stress and regulating emotions, leading to improved health outcomes.

4. **Perception and Pain**

Emotions influence how we perceive physical sensations, including pain. Negative emotions can amplify pain, while positive emotions can help diminish its impact. This is why mindfulness and cognitive behavioral therapy, which focus on reinterpreting emotional and physical experiences, can improve health outcomes.

5. **Social and Emotional Contexts**

Emotional well-being is tied to social interactions and support. Positive emotional experiences within social contexts can strengthen immune function and improve illness recovery, while loneliness or emotional neglect can have the opposite effect.

**Practical Implications:**

Barrett's insights suggest that cultivating emotional awareness and improving emotional regulation can enhance physical health. Strategies such as mindfulness, expanding emotional vocabulary, and engaging in supportive social relationships can help maintain a healthier body budget and improve overall well-being.

# The Connection between Positive Psychology and Nursing:

Positive psychology and nursing share a common goal promoting health and well-being. Both fields emphasize the importance of addressing the whole person rather than just treating specific health problems. Positive psychology research has shown that positive emotions can have a significant impact on physical health, such as improving immune function and reducing the risk of chronic disease (Fredrickson, 2013). Thus, nursing interventions that promote positive emotions can contribute to overall health and well-being.

One key principle of New Thought is the belief in the power of the mind to influence the body. Research in psychoneuroimmunology, which studies the interactions between the mind, the nervous system, and the immune system, has supported this idea. Studies have shown that positive emotions and attitudes can improve immune function, while negative emotions and stress can suppress it (Segerstrom & Miller, 2004).

One significant takeaway from this exploration is that the mind and body are interconnected. Numerous studies have documented this connection, and the evidence affirms that our thoughts and emotions can significantly impact our physical health (Lipton, 2015; Segerstrom & Miller, 2004). Additionally, positive thought and intention have been linked to improved patient outcomes, including pain management, decreased anxiety, and shorter hospital stays.

The concept of presentiment affirms that current physiological states are linked to imminent future experiences. Specifically, when these future experiences involve emotional stimuli—such as viewing photographs with varying emotional content—this connection is hypothesized to manifest as a present-time activation of the autonomic nervous system. (Radin, D. 2004).

This proves that an individual's thoughts and emotions can significantly impact their physical health and well-being, regardless of the stimuli.

## Positive Relationships lead to Healthier Living.

Cultivating positive relationships and experiences can also contribute to overall happiness and well-being. Focusing on positive emotions, strengths, and virtues can lead to greater happiness and well-being. Negative emotions and experiences should not be ignored but transformed into positive ones through reframing and cognitive reappraisal. Encouraging positive thoughts and emotions can improve health outcomes and enhance patient satisfaction.

The mind has a significant impact on the body. Positive thoughts and emotions can improve physical health, and visualization and affirmations can enhance well-being. The mind and body are interconnected. Stress, negative emotions, and beliefs can have detrimental effects on physical health. Practices that promote relaxation and positive emotions can enhance physical health.

Positive psychology emphasizes focusing on positive emotions, strengths, and virtues to promote happiness and well-being. Negative experiences and emotions should be transformed into positive ones through reframing and cognitive reappraisal. Cultivating positive relationships and experiences is also crucial for overall happiness and well-being.

## Emotions in Nursing Practice & Healthcare

Nurses should incorporate positive psychology principles to promote positive emotions, thoughts, and behaviors. The new nursing theory emphasizes the power of thoughts and positive emotions on health and healing. The mind-body connection is a core principle of this theory, highlighting the interconnectedness between mental and physical health. The theory also advocates using meditation, mindfulness, and positive thinking to enhance this connection.

In healthcare, patients often focus on their physical symptoms, but it is essential to understand that emotions and thoughts also play a significant role in overall health and healing. Negative thoughts and defeatist ideations can be sincerely held and challenging to overcome, but with the right techniques and practices, patients can learn to acknowledge and challenge them.

In addition to these practices, patient education is crucial for creating lasting change. Nurses can play a significant role in teaching patients about the power of positive thoughts and emotions and the potential of the quantum world through thought, emotion, and positive love-based intention. This education can include information about the interconnectedness of all things and how patients can cultivate positive energy through self-care practices, such as exercise, healthy eating, and social support.

## Emotions, Prayer, and Healing:

Another way in which prayer may affect reality on a subatomic level is through the power of emotion. Emotions are energy in motion and can create a coherent field of energy that influences the behavior of subatomic particles. Positive emotions, such as love and gratitude, have been shown to have a measurable effect on physical systems, while negative emotions, such as fear and anger, can have a detrimental effect.

The relationship between prayer and quantum physics is a complex and multifaceted topic, and more research is needed to fully understand the mechanisms by which prayer may affect reality on a subatomic level. However, quantum physics observations suggest that our thoughts and emotions can have a powerful influence on the physical world and that prayer may be a powerful tool for harnessing this influence.

The relationship between prayer and quantum physics is an exciting and rapidly evolving study area. The power of the mind and emotions to affect reality on a subatomic level is a concept that has far-reaching implications for both science and spirituality. As we continue to explore the mysteries of the quantum world, we may gain new insights into the nature of reality and our place in the universe.

Greg Braden, an American author and speaker, has explored the relationship between prayer and quantum physics for several years. In his book "The Divine Matrix: Bridging Time, Space, Miracles, and Belief," Braden presents evidence that affirms prayer can influence our reality on a subatomic level. Braden argues that understanding the connection between prayer and quantum physics could lead to a greater understanding of the universe and our place in it.

At the heart of Braden's argument is the concept of the "Divine Matrix." This matrix is an energy field that connects all things in the universe. According to Braden, this matrix is the source of all creation and the key to understanding the power of prayer. In the book, he writes:

"The Divine Matrix is the container that holds the universe, the bridge between all things, and the mirror that shows us what we have created. It is everything we have ever known, everything we will ever know, and everything we have yet to imagine."

Braden believes that by tapping into the Divine Matrix through prayer, we can influence the physical world around us. He argues that prayer is not just a request for divine intervention but rather a way to align our thoughts and emotions with the underlying energy of the universe. This alignment creates a resonance between our thoughts and the quantum field, which can then manifest in the physical world.

Braden's ideas are not without scientific support. In recent years, scientists have made several discoveries that support the notion that our thoughts and emotions can influence the physical world. One such discovery is the observer effect, a principle in quantum physics that states that observation can change the behavior of subatomic particles. As physicist John Wheeler once said, "We make the universe by observing it."

Another scientific principle supporting Braden's ideas is quantum entanglement. This principle affirms that particles can become linked together so that the state of one particle can affect the state of another particle, regardless of the distance between them. This affirms a kind of interconnectedness between all things in the universe, which could support the idea of the Divine Matrix.

In his book, Braden also cites several studies that suggest prayer can have a real effect on the physical world. Dr. Randolph Byrd, a cardiologist at San Francisco General Hospital, conducted one such study. In the study, patients in the cardiac care unit were randomly assigned to either a group that received prayer from a group of Christians or a control group that did not receive prayer. The study found that the patients who received prayer had fewer complications and required fewer medications than those in the control group.

Braden's work has been met with some criticism from the scientific community. Some scientists argue that the effects of prayer could simply be due to the placebo effect or other psychological factors. However, Braden argues that the placebo effect is still a real effect and that the power of prayer could still be harnessed for healing and other purposes.

In conclusion, Greg Braden's exploration into the connection between prayer and quantum physics is a fascinating topic that has the potential to shed new light on our understanding of the universe. Braden's ideas are supported by scientific principles such as the observer effect and quantum entanglement, as well as by real-world studies that suggest prayer can have a real effect on the physical world. Whether or not one believes in the power of prayer, Braden's work offers an intriguing perspective on the nature of reality and our place in it. As he writes in "The Divine Matrix":

"Through the eyes of quantum physics, we see ourselves and our world differently. We are more than we have ever imagined, and we are closer to the divine than we have ever known."

## The Emotion of Love and Healing:

Furthermore, many scientists have observed the effects of positive emotions such as love on the quantum level. In the book "The Holographic Universe," author Michael Talbot writes, "The holographic model affirms that the physical universe is not a concrete reality but is, instead, a kind of illusion, or more accurately, a projection of a higher-dimensional reality which cannot be perceived in normal waking consciousness." This higher-dimensional reality, which Talbot refers to as the "implicate order," is said to be influenced by consciousness, particularly positive emotions such as love.

Several studies have shown that positive emotions such as love and compassion can have a measurable effect on the physical world. In one study conducted by the HeartMath Institute, researchers found that individuals who focused on feelings of love and appreciation had a measurable effect on the surrounding environment. The study found that positive emotions has a direct impact on the heart's electromagnetic field, which in turn affected the physical world around the individual.

In addition, research has shown that positive emotions such as love and compassion can have a beneficial effect on the human body. Studies have found that individuals who regularly practice positive emotions such as gratitude, forgiveness, and compassion have a lower risk of developing chronic illnesses such as heart disease, diabetes, and depression. This may be because positive emotions have been shown to reduce stress and inflammation in the body, both of which are contributing factors to chronic illness.

In conclusion, the concept of love as a universal force is gaining more attention in the scientific community. Evidence affirms that positive emotions such as love and compassion have a measurable effect on the quantum level and can also have a beneficial effect on the human body. The unified field theory and quantum physics provide a framework for understanding the relationship between love and the universe. The implications of this relationship are far-reaching and offer the potential for a more harmonious and connected existence for all.

Our emotions, feelings, and beliefs are crucial in communicating with the unified field of love. As we have previously discussed, the field of energy is what connects us to everything and all possibilities all at once, allowing the manifestation of desired outcomes. In order to effectively communicate with this field, it is crucial to understand that our thoughts and emotions have a vibrational frequency that can influence the energy around us.

The principles of quantum physics suggest that everything in the universe comprises energy and that all energy is connected. This means that our thoughts and emotions can influence the energy around us and, in turn, affect the outcomes we experience.

# Conclusion

"Our emotions, feelings, and beliefs are how we communicate with the unified field of love. This field of energy connects us to everything and all possibilities all at once, allowing the manifestation of desired outcomes in and out of the world of nursing." (Dossey, 2013, p. 67)

Negative thoughts and emotions can significantly impact mental and physical health. However, by acknowledging these thoughts and purposefully changing our perspective, we can overcome them and focus on solutions and desired outcomes. Nurses can play a crucial role in helping patients develop a positive mindset by educating them on techniques to overcome negative thoughts and improve their mental and physical well-being. By embracing the power of positive thinking, we can create a more optimistic and fulfilling life.

Our emotions, feelings, and beliefs are how we communicate with the unified field of love and access its unlimited potential. As discussed earlier, the quantum nursing theory proposes that the universe comprises energy, frequency, and vibrations and that all things are interconnected through this unified field.

Our thoughts and emotions carry their own vibrations and frequencies. When we align them with the high frequency of love, we create a powerful resonance that attracts similar frequencies and vibrations in our environment. This is known as the law of attraction, and it operates based on the principle that like attracts like.

As Dr. Bruce Lipton states in his book The Biology of Belief, our beliefs and thoughts constantly shape our reality. He writes, "The moment you change your perception is the moment you rewrite the chemistry of your body" (Lipton, 2005, p. 167). This highlights the power of our thoughts and beliefs to affect our physical bodies and environment.

When we focus our thoughts and emotions on the desired outcomes, we message the unified field of love that we are ready to receive them. The field responds by reflecting back to us the vibrations and frequencies that match our desires, and this creates a feedback loop of manifestation.

In the context of nursing, this means that we can use our thoughts, emotions, and beliefs to manifest the outcomes we want for our patients and ourselves. For instance, if we want to create a healing environment for our patients, we can cultivate feelings of love, compassion, and gratitude and focus our thoughts on the positive outcomes we want to see. Doing so sends a powerful signal to the unified field of love that attracts the frequencies and vibrations that align with our intentions.

Moreover, our thoughts and emotions also affect the energy field of those around us, including our patients. As nurses, we have the power to influence the energy field of our patients through our thoughts, emotions, and intentions. Creating a positive and loving environment can help our patients heal faster and feel more empowered in their recovery process.

In conclusion, the quantum nursing theory emphasizes the importance of understanding the interconnectedness of all things and the role of our thoughts, emotions, and beliefs in manifesting desired outcomes. By aligning ourselves with the high frequency of love and using it as a means of communication with the unified field, we can tap into its unlimited potential and create positive change in the world of nursing and beyond.

## References

Fredrickson, B. L. (2013). Positive emotions broaden and build. In Advances in experimental social psychology (Vol. 47, pp. 1-53). Academic Press.

Segerstrom SC, Miller GE. Psychological stress and the human immune system: a meta-analytic study of 30 years of inquiry. Psychol Bull. 2004 Jul;130(4):601-30. doi: 10.1037/0033-2909.130.4.601. PMID: 15250815; PMCID: PMC1361287.

Radin, D. 2004. Electrodermal presentiments of future emotions. Journal of Scientific Exploration, 18(2), 253–273.

Koob GF. The dark side of emotion: The addiction perspective. *Eur J Pharmacol.* 2015;753:73-87. doi:10.1016/j.ejphar.2014.11.044

# Chapter 8: The Role of Nutrition in Healthcare & Nursing

Nutrition and exercise are essential for your physical and mental health. The New Nursing Theory of the Power of Love and Holistic Health is a comprehensive theory that considers various nursing philosophies and integrates them with modern scientific research to provide a holistic approach to healthcare. This theory acknowledges the importance of the mind-body-spirit connection and the impact of love, nutrition, and positive energy on an individual's health and well-being.

The theory recognizes the importance of nutrition in promoting health and well-being. It emphasizes the need for nurses to provide guidance and education on healthy eating habits to patients and their families. The theory also recognizes the importance of environmental factors in promoting health and emphasizes the need for nurses to create safe and healthy environments for patients.

Nutrition is a fundamental component of healthcare. Proper nutrition supports optimal physical and emotional health and can prevent and manage many health conditions. Nutrition and Lifestyle Modifications emphasize the importance of a healthy diet, exercise, and lifestyle modifications in promoting optimal health. Many studies on the impact of nutrition and lifestyle modifications on chronic disease management and prevention have explored the effects of nutrition on patient outcomes in the context of the new nursing theory-based care.

Nutrition plays a critical role in nursing practice. It is significant in promoting health and preventing disease. Proper nutrition can improve patient outcomes and enhance the overall quality of care.

# Diet and Lifestyle

Diet and lifestyle choices are major contributors to many medical problems and have a significant impact on the healthcare system. In recent years, there has been a growing body of research demonstrating the link between diet, lifestyle, and chronic diseases such as obesity, type 2 diabetes, cardiovascular disease, and cancer.

In the United States, chronic diseases account for more than 80% of all healthcare spending, and the costs associated with these diseases are projected to reach $6 trillion by 2030. Chronic diseases, such as heart disease, stroke, diabetes, and certain types of cancer, are largely preventable. This is a significant burden on the healthcare system, and it is clear that addressing the root causes of chronic diseases, such as diet and lifestyle factors, could have a significant impact on reducing healthcare costs and improving overall health outcomes.

Research has shown that dietary factors play a key role in developing and managing chronic diseases. For example, diets high in saturated fat added sugars, and processed foods have been linked to an increased risk of heart disease and type 2 diabetes. On the other hand, diets rich in fruits, vegetables, whole grains, and lean protein sources have been associated with a reduced risk of chronic diseases.

Poor diet, characterized by excessive consumption of highly processed and energy-dense foods, is a leading risk factor for chronic diseases. These foods are rich in saturated and trans fats, added sugars, and sodium while being low in fiber, vitamins, and minerals. Additionally, low intake of fruits, vegetables, whole grains, and lean protein sources, such as fish and nuts, is associated with an increased risk of chronic diseases. According to the World Health Organization, over 60% of all deaths worldwide are caused by chronic diseases, and this number is expected to continue to rise in the coming years.

Lifestyle factors, such as physical inactivity, smoking, excessive alcohol consumption, and poor sleep quality, also contribute to the development of chronic diseases. Physical inactivity is a major risk factor for heart disease, stroke, and type 2 diabetes. Smoking is the leading cause of preventable death worldwide and is a major risk factor for several types of cancer. Excessive alcohol consumption is associated with liver disease, cancer, and other health problems. Poor sleep quality has been linked to obesity, type 2 diabetes, and cardiovascular disease.

The burden of chronic diseases on the healthcare system is significant. Chronic diseases are the leading cause of hospitalization and emergency department visits in the United States. They also require long-term management and treatment, which can be costly. In addition to the direct healthcare costs, chronic diseases also impose a substantial economic burden through lost productivity and decreased quality of life.

Preventive measures, such as dietary and lifestyle modifications, can significantly reduce the risk of chronic diseases and their associated healthcare costs. Therefore, healthcare providers need to incorporate nutrition and lifestyle counseling into their practice. However, as mentioned earlier, medical doctors receive very little training in nutrition and often lack the knowledge and skills to counsel patients on dietary and lifestyle modifications effectively.

In addition to diet, physical activity is also a critical factor in preventing and managing chronic diseases. Lack of physical activity has been linked to an increased risk of obesity, heart disease, and type 2 diabetes. On the other hand, regular exercise has been shown to improve cardiovascular health, reduce the risk of chronic diseases, and improve overall quality of life.

Smoking is another major contributor to chronic diseases and is responsible for approximately 480,000 deaths each year in the United States alone. Quitting smoking is one of the most effective ways to reduce the risk of chronic diseases and improve overall health outcomes.

Excessive alcohol consumption is one major contributor to chronic diseases, including liver disease, certain types of cancer, and cardiovascular disease. It is recommended that adults consume alcohol in moderation, which is defined as up to one drink per day for women and up to two drinks per day for men.

Nutrition is a crucial factor in maintaining good health. The food we eat provide the energy and nutrients our bodies need to function optimally. Good nutrition is essential for healthy growth and development, disease prevention, and overall well-being. This chapter will discuss the importance of nutrition in health, including the role of macronutrients and micronutrients, the impact of nutrition on chronic diseases, and the importance of a balanced diet.

Nutrition and exercise can help you create a healing environment for patients, and they can also:

- **Improve your health**

A healthy diet and regular exercise can help reduce your risk of chronic diseases like diabetes, heart disease, high blood pressure, stroke, and some cancers. They can also help you manage your weight, boost energy levels, and improve your memory and concentration.

- **Improve your mental health**

Nutrition and exercise can help improve your mood and behavior, and stimulate the release of neurotransmitters that enhance your pleasure, motivation, and learning.

- **Improve your immune system**

A diet high in fruits and vegetables, combined with regular physical activity, can help improve your immune function.

- **Prevent bone diseases**

Weight-bearing exercise and a diet with enough calcium can help prevent osteoporosis.

- **Slow down aging**

A healthy diet and regular exercise can help slow down the process of aging.

- **Save money on healthcare**

By preventing disease and staying healthy, you can spend less on healthcare in the long term.

Here are some tips for eating well and staying active:

- **Drink enough fluids**

Drink about 6-8 cups of water daily to help prevent and treat constipation.

- **Eat enough calcium**

Calcium is important for strong bones and teeth, especially during periods of rapid growth like childhood and adolescence. Good sources of calcium include dairy products, fortified plant-based alternatives, and leafy green vegetables.

- **Eat leafy greens**

Leafy greens contain nitrates that convert to nitric oxide, which can improve blood flow during exercise.

# The Role of Micronutrients

Micronutrients are the nutrients we need in smaller amounts, including vitamins and minerals. They are essential for maintaining proper bodily functions, such as immune function, blood clotting, and bone health. A deficiency in micronutrients can lead to a range of health problems, including anamia, osteoporosis, and weakened immune function.

Fruits and vegetables are excellent sources of micronutrients, including vitamins A, C, and K, as well as minerals such as potassium, magnesium, and calcium. A diet rich in fruits and vegetables has been linked to a lower risk of chronic diseases such as heart disease, cancer, and diabetes.

# Impact of Nutrition on Chronic Diseases

Chronic diseases such as heart disease, cancer, and diabetes are the leading causes of death worldwide. Nutrition plays a crucial role in the prevention and management of chronic diseases. A diet high in saturated and trans fats, sugar, and salt is linked to an increased risk of chronic diseases, while a diet rich in fruits, vegetables, whole grains, and lean proteins is associated with a lower risk.

For example, a diet high in red meat is associated with an increased risk of colorectal cancer, while a diet high in fruits and vegetables has been linked to a lower risk. High salt intake is associated with an increased risk of high blood pressure, while a diet low in sodium and high in potassium has been linked to a lower risk.

### Importance of a Balanced Diet

A balanced diet is essential for optimal health. It should include a variety of fruits and vegetables, whole grains, lean proteins, and healthy fats. Eating a balanced diet ensures that we get all the essential nutrients our bodies need, including macronutrients, micronutrients, and phytochemicals.

Phytochemicals are natural compounds found in plant-based foods that have health benefits beyond basic nutrition. For example, lycopene, a phytochemical found in tomatoes, is associated with a lower risk of prostate cancer.

A balanced diet also helps to maintain a healthy weight and reduce the risk of chronic diseases. Eating a diet high in fruits, vegetables, and whole grains can help to lower cholesterol levels and blood pressure, reducing the risk of heart disease. A diet low in saturated and trans fats can help to lower the risk of obesity and type 2 diabetes.

## Biohacking and Optimal Health

**Biohacking** refers to the practice of making systematic, science-informed interventions to one's biology with the aim of improving health, performance, and well-being. It encompasses a broad spectrum of approaches, ranging from simple lifestyle modifications, such as optimizing diet and exercise, to advanced interventions like the use of wearable technology, nootropics, genetic editing, and other experimental tools. Biohacking is often categorized into do-it-yourself (DIY) experimentation, supported by personal monitoring and data analysis, and professionally guided approaches rooted in clinical research.

**Optimal Health** is a dynamic state of physical, mental, emotional, and social well-being achieved through balanced and sustainable practices and also promotes vitality, resilience, and longevity. It is characterized by the efficient functioning of the body and mind, the absence of disease or chronic conditions, and the ability to adapt to life's stressors while maintaining overall quality of life. Optimal health emphasizes not merely the absence of illness but the cultivation of a holistic state of thriving across multiple dimensions of human experience.

These concepts often intersect in the context of contemporary health science, as biohacking strategies are increasingly employed to achieve and sustain optimal health through evidence-based methods and personalized health interventions.

Brendon Burchard, Ben Greenfield, and Tim Ferriss have made significant contributions to biohacking and optimal health, though their approaches vary slightly based on their individual expertise and perspectives.

**Brendon Burchard**

Brendon Burchard primarily focuses on personal performance and high-energy living, with an emphasis on creating habits that support physical, mental, and emotional well-being. His works, such as *High-Performance Habits*, outline strategies for maximizing energy and vitality, foundational to optimal health. Key aspects include:

**Nutrition:** Advocating for a balanced diet that fuels energy and mental clarity.

**Physical Activity:** Encouraging consistent exercise to enhance mood, focus, and stamina.

**Mindfulness Practices:** Promoting meditation and mindfulness to manage stress and maintain emotional resilience.

**Sleep Hygiene:** Highlighting the importance of restorative sleep for sustained performance and longevity.

## Ben Greenfield

Ben Greenfield is a prominent voice in biohacking, merging traditional health principles with cutting-edge science. His works, such as *Boundless* and *Beyond Training*, delve deep into optimizing human biology for peak performance and longevity. His approach includes:

**Nutrition:** Advocating for nutrient-dense, whole foods, and intermittent fasting to enhance metabolic health. He often discusses the benefits of ketogenic and paleo diets.

**Exercise:** Introducing advanced training methods, like high-intensity interval training (HIIT), and the strategic use of recovery protocols, such as cryotherapy and infrared saunas.

**Supplements and Biohacking Tools:** Exploring the use of nootropics, adaptogens, and wearable tech to monitor and improve health metrics.

**Holistic Practices:** Stressing the importance of mental and spiritual health through practices like cold exposure, grounding, and gratitude journaling.

## Tim Ferriss

Tim Ferriss, known for *the 4-Hour Body* and *Tools of Titans*, is a pioneer in self-experimentation, offering practical and unconventional hacks for optimizing health and performance. His approach includes:

**Dietary Experiments:** Popular methods like the slow-carb diet, cyclic ketogenic diets, and precise caloric restrictions are useful to achieve fat loss and energy optimization.

**Sleep Optimization:** Introducing polyphasic sleep patterns and other sleep hacks to enhance recovery and cognitive performance.

**Micro habits:** Encouraging small, impactful changes that yield significant health and performance improvements, such as starting the day with a protein-rich meal or using light therapy.

**Data-Driven Approach:** Advocating for the use of wearable tech, apps, and other tracking systems to gather insights and make informed decisions about health and fitness routines.

Across their works, there are several unifying themes:

**Individualization:** Tailoring health and lifestyle practices to fit personal needs and goals.

**Science-Backed Methods:** Integrating evidence-based strategies alongside self-experimentation.

**Holistic Focus:** Addressing not only physical health but also mental, emotional, and spiritual well-being.

**Empowerment through Education:** Encouraging individuals to take charge of their health through informed decisions and habit-building.

These authors provide actionable advice for improving nutrition, energy levels, and overall health, offering diverse yet complementary insights into biohacking and lifestyle transformation.

## FDA's Role in the Safety of the American Food Supply

The issue of corruption and the revolving door between private and public firms influencing regulations is complex and contentious. In the context of the FDA and the American food supply, it has been widely reported that the agency has been heavily influenced by industry interests, leading to a lack of effective regulation and oversight.

*The regulation of food and consumer products by the U.S. Food and Drug Administration (FDA) has been a subject of ongoing debate, particularly regarding the approval of certain additives and substances that are restricted or banned in other countries, such as those in the European Union. Research has raised concerns about the potential effects of certain food additives and chemicals on cognitive function, metabolic processes, and overall well-being. Some studies suggest that exposure to these substances may influence neurological activity, potentially affecting clarity of thought and cognitive performance. Given that mental clarity and cognitive function play a crucial role in decision-making, emotional regulation, and overall quality of life, the inclusion of such substances in the food supply warrants further scrutiny.*

*Furthermore, emerging research in nutritional epigenetics indicates that dietary habits may play a significant role in the development of certain health conditions previously considered hereditary. This demonstrates that generational dietary patterns could contribute to the prevalence of metabolic and neurological disorders, emphasizing the importance of nutrition education for healthcare providers. By incorporating evidence-based nutritional guidance into patient care, practitioners may better support individuals in making informed dietary choices that promote cognitive and metabolic health.*

The Food and Drug Administration (FDA) is a regulatory agency tasked with ensuring the safety and efficacy of food, drugs, and medical devices in the United States. However, there are growing concerns that the FDA is failing in its role to keep the American food supply optimal for promoting optimal health in the American diet.

One of the primary concerns is the FDA's reliance on the food industry to conduct its own safety testing. This self-regulation system allows the food industry to operate with minimal oversight, resulting in numerous instances of contaminated or adulterated food entering the food supply. For example, the recent outbreaks of *E. coli* in romaine lettuce and salmonella in eggs highlight the inadequacy of the current regulatory system.

Another rising issue is the FDA's lack of oversight over certain food industry aspects, such as genetically modified organisms (GMOs). Despite mounting evidence of the potential health risks associated with GMOs, the FDA has not taken steps to require labeling or limit the use of these products in the food supply.

Additionally, the FDA's standards for what is considered safe for consumption are often outdated and based on flawed research. For example, the FDA's daily recommended values for nutrients such as vitamin D and calcium have been criticized for being too low and not reflective of the latest research on optimal nutrient intake.

Another area of concern is the revolving door between industry and government. Many high-level FDA officials have previously worked for or have strong ties to the industries they are meant to regulate. This can lead to a bias in favor of industry interests and a lack of effective regulation.

Another issue is the regulatory capture of the FDA by industry. This occurs when industry interests become so influential that the FDA becomes a tool for promoting those interests rather than protecting public health. This can lead to lax regulation and oversight, as well as a lack of enforcement against industry violations.

The issue of corruption and industry influence is further complicated by the role of lobbyists and campaign contributions. Lobbyists can exert significant influence on government officials and policymakers, often working to promote the interests of their clients. Campaign contributions can also have a significant impact, with politicians often being more responsive to the interests of their donors than to the needs of the general public.

In the context of nutrition and healthcare, the issue of industry influence on the FDA and other regulatory bodies has serious consequences. Many health experts argue that the standard American diet is heavily influenced by industry interests, with the focus on processed foods and high-calorie, low-nutrient options.

Furthermore, the lack of effective regulation and oversight can lead to dangerous levels of contaminants and additives in food products, as well as misleading or false claims about their health benefits. This can have severe implications for public health, particularly in vulnerable populations such as children and the elderly.

One of the main areas of concern is the FDA's reliance on industry-funded research and data. This can create conflicts of interest, with industry representatives having a strong influence on the agency's decisions. In addition, the FDA often relies on self-regulation by industry, which can lead to a lack of transparency and accountability.

Overall, the issue of corruption and industry influence on the FDA and other regulatory bodies is a significant concern for public health and the American food supply. While the FDA plays a critical role in ensuring the safety of the American food supply, there are numerous concerns that it fails to promote optimal health in the American diet. The agency must strengthen its regulatory processes, increase transparency and accountability, and prioritize public health over industry interests. Addressing this issue will require a concerted effort by government officials, industry representatives, and concerned citizens to promote transparency, accountability, and effective regulation.

## The Role of Nutrition in Healthcare

The role of nutrition in healthcare has gained increasing attention in recent years, as studies have shown the significant impact that diet can have on preventing and treating chronic diseases. However, despite this growing understanding of the importance of nutrition, medical doctors continue to receive minimal training in nutritional approaches to therapeutic interventions.

The lack of nutrition education in medical schools has been well-documented. A study published in the American Journal of Clinical Nutrition found that medical students receive an average of just 19.6 hours of nutrition education across their entire medical school curriculum. This is in stark contrast to the 25 to 30 hours of pharmacology that medical students typically receive.

The consequences of this lack of education are significant. Without a solid understanding of the role of nutrition in disease prevention and treatment, doctors may miss critical opportunities to help their patients make dietary changes that could significantly improve their health outcomes. A study published in the Journal of the American Medical Association found that only 14% of physicians feel adequately trained to provide nutritional counseling to their patients.

In addition, doctors may rely too heavily on pharmaceutical interventions to manage chronic conditions rather than exploring the potential benefits of dietary changes. This can lead to over-prescribing of medications, which can have significant side effects and may not address the root cause of the patient's health issues.

Fortunately, efforts are underway to address this issue. Medical schools are beginning to recognize the importance of nutrition education and are incorporating it into their curricula. In addition, professional organizations such as the American Medical Association and the Academy of Nutrition and Dietetics are working to increase awareness of the importance of nutrition education for medical professionals.

Healthcare professionals need to recognize nutrition's crucial role in promoting optimal health outcomes for their patients, providing adequate nutrition education for medical professionals, and encouraging a focus on dietary interventions.

While nutrition plays a critical role in overall health and disease prevention, medical doctors are often poorly trained in this area. Medical education has traditionally focused on the diagnosis and treatment of diseases rather than prevention through healthy lifestyles and nutrition. This lack of emphasis on nutrition education in medical schools has contributed to a healthcare system that is reactive rather than proactive and has led to a growing need for nutrition experts in healthcare.

A study published in the Journal of the American College of Nutrition found that medical students receive an average of just 23.9 hours of nutrition education throughout their four years of medical school, far less than the 25 to 30 hours recommended by the National Academy of Sciences. Furthermore, the same study found that 71% of medical schools failed to meet the minimum recommended hours of nutrition education.

The lack of emphasis on nutrition education in medical schools can have several negative consequences for patients. For example, doctors may be less likely to recognize the role that nutrition plays in the prevention and management of chronic diseases such as obesity, type 2 diabetes, and heart disease. They may also be less likely to recommend dietary changes to patients or may provide incorrect or outdated nutritional advice.

The problem of inadequate nutrition education in medical schools is further compounded by the influence of the pharmaceutical and food industries. These industries have significant financial interests in maintaining the status quo, which includes a healthcare system that relies on pharmaceutical interventions and processed foods rather than prevention and whole-food-based interventions.

The pharmaceutical industry, for example, has a vested interest in promoting drugs as the primary solution for disease management. This leads to a focus on treating symptoms rather than addressing underlying causes, such as poor nutrition. Additionally, pharmaceutical companies often sponsor medical schools and research, creating conflicts of interest and influencing the curriculum and research priorities.

The food industry also significantly influences the healthcare system, shaping dietary guidelines and policies. Food companies have a vested interest in promoting processed foods and sugary beverages, which contribute to chronic diseases. They also have a history of funding research that promotes their products and downplays their negative health effects.

In conclusion, the lack of emphasis on nutrition education in medical schools is a significant problem that has negative consequences for patients. Inadequate training in nutrition can lead to incorrect or outdated nutritional advice, a focus on treating symptoms rather than underlying causes, and an over-reliance on pharmaceutical interventions. Additionally, the influence of the pharmaceutical and food industries further compounds the problem. Medical schools and the healthcare system as a whole must prioritize nutrition education to serve patients better and promote overall health and wellness.

# Nutrition and Its Role in Nursing Practice

Nutrition is a crucial component of health and wellness. It plays a key role in preventing and managing chronic diseases, such as obesity, diabetes, and heart disease. Proper nutrition is also essential for wound healing, immune function, and maintaining healthy skin and hair.

In nursing practice, proper nutrition is critical for promoting health and preventing disease. Nurses play a vital role in promoting proper nutrition and educating patients about healthy eating habits. They also monitor patients' nutritional status and make recommendations for dietary changes as needed.

Poor nutrition can have significant negative impacts on patient outcomes. Malnutrition can lead to weakened immune systems, delayed wound healing, and increased risk of infections. In older adults, malnutrition can lead to frailty and an increased risk of falls. In children, poor nutrition can lead to developmental delays and growth issues.

## Principles of Nutrition in Nursing Practice

The principles of nutrition in nursing practice focus on understanding and applying dietary knowledge to promote health, prevent disease, and manage illnesses. These principles are rooted in the science of human physiology, metabolism, and the role of nutrients in maintaining bodily functions. Key principles include:

1. **Adequacy:** Ensuring the diet provides sufficient nutrients, including carbohydrates, proteins, fats, vitamins, and minerals, to meet the individual's physiological needs.

2. **Balance:** Combining different food groups in appropriate proportions to maintain health and avoid nutrient deficiencies or excesses.

3. **Calorie Control:** Regulating energy intake to align with an individual's energy expenditure, supporting healthy weight maintenance and metabolic function.

4. **Nutrient Density:** Prioritizing foods that are rich in essential nutrients relative to their calorie content, promoting better health outcomes.

5. **Variety:** Including diverse foods in the diet to ensure a comprehensive intake of nutrients and to reduce the risk of developing nutrient deficiencies.

6. **Moderation:** Avoiding overconsumption of any particular food or nutrient, especially those associated with adverse health effects, like saturated fats, added sugars, and sodium.

## Importance of Nutrition in Nursing Practice

Nutrition is a cornerstone of nursing practice, significantly impacting patient outcomes and overall well-being. Its importance is multifaceted:

1. **Health Promotion and Disease Prevention:**

    - Nurses play a critical role in educating patients about healthy eating patterns to prevent chronic diseases such as diabetes, cardiovascular diseases, and obesity.

    - Nutritional counseling can support lifelong wellness and reduce the risk of malnutrition.

2. **Management of Illness:**

- Adequate nutrition is essential in recovery from surgeries, infections, and illnesses. For instance, protein supports wound healing, while certain diets can manage conditions like renal failure or diabetes.

- Specialized diets, such as low-sodium or high-fiber diets, are tailored to manage specific health conditions.

3. **Support for Vulnerable Populations:**

    - Nurses assess and address nutritional needs in vulnerable groups, including children, the elderly, pregnant women, and individuals with chronic diseases or disabilities.

    - Identifying and intervening in cases of malnutrition or food insecurity is an integral part of nursing care.

4. **Patient Education and Advocacy:**

    - Nurses educate patients and families about meal planning, dietary modifications, and the impact of nutrition on health.

    - They advocate for policy changes and institutional practices that ensure access to nutritious food, especially in clinical or community settings.

5. **Interdisciplinary Collaboration:**

    - Nurses often collaborate with dietitians, physicians, and other healthcare professionals to develop and implement individualized nutrition care plans.

- They monitor patient progress, ensuring adherence to nutritional interventions and adjusting plans as needed.

By integrating the principles of nutrition into practice, nurses enhance their ability to provide holistic care, support healing processes, and improve the quality of life for their patients.

## The Role of Nutrition in Disease Prevention

Here are some additional examples of the role of nutrition in disease prevention:

**Cardiovascular disease:** A diet high in saturated and trans fats, cholesterol, and sodium is a major risk factor for heart disease. On the other hand, a diet rich in fruits, vegetables, whole grains, nuts, and healthy fats like omega-3s can help prevent heart disease by lowering blood pressure, reducing inflammation, and improving cholesterol levels.

**Type 2 diabetes:** A diet high in sugar and refined carbohydrates can increase the risk of developing type 2 diabetes. Eating a diet rich in fiber, whole grains, and healthy fats can help regulate blood sugar levels and reduce the risk of developing diabetes.

**Cancer:** Studies have shown that certain nutrients and compounds found in fruits, vegetables, and whole grains can help reduce the risk of cancer. For example, cruciferous vegetables like broccoli and cauliflower contain sulforaphane, which has been shown to have anti-cancer properties.

**Osteoporosis:** Adequate calcium and vitamin D intake is essential for maintaining strong bones and reducing the risk of osteoporosis. Foods like dairy products, leafy green vegetables, and fortified cereals can provide these essential nutrients.

Overall, a balanced and varied diet that includes a variety of whole foods is key for disease prevention. In addition, avoiding processed and high-fat foods, limiting sugar and alcohol intake, and maintaining a healthy weight can also help reduce the risk of chronic diseases.

## Nutrition and the Mind-Gut Connection

Nutrition plays a critical role in maintaining cognitive function and overall wellness. The food we eat not only provides energy for the body but also nutrients that are necessary for proper brain function. The mind-gut connection, as described by Dr. Ben Greenfield in his book Boundless, emphasizes the importance of a healthy gut microbiome for mental and physical health.

Research has shown that the gut microbiome is key in regulating brain function and behavior, including mood, anxiety, and cognition. The gut-brain axis is a bidirectional communication pathway between the gut and the central nervous system, which is essential for maintaining homeostasis in the body. Thus, it is becoming clear that maintaining a healthy microbiome is crucial to having a healthy brain across the lifespan from cradle to grave. Studies have demonstrated that changes in the gut microbiome can affect brain function, leading to a range of neuropsychiatric disorders, i.e., there is growing evidence that the gut microbiota and nutrition have an impact on the onset and course of psychiatric disorders.

Nutrition plays a critical role in maintaining a healthy gut microbiome. A diet that is high in fiber, fruits, and vegetables has been shown to promote the growth of beneficial gut bacteria, while a diet that is high in sugar and saturated fats can lead to an overgrowth of harmful bacteria. In addition to the types of foods we eat, the timing of our meals and the frequency of our eating can also affect the gut microbiome.

Research has also shown that specific nutrients can support cognitive function and brain health. For example, omega-3 fatty acids, which are found in fatty fish, nuts, and seeds, have been shown to improve cognitive function and reduce the risk of cognitive decline. B vitamins, such as folate and vitamin B12, are essential for brain function and are found in leafy green vegetables, legumes, and fortified cereals.

Incorporating a healthy diet and lifestyle habits can have a significant impact on cognitive function and overall wellness. Nursing professionals can play a crucial role in educating patients about the importance of nutrition and the mind-gut connection. By promoting a healthy diet and lifestyle habits, nurses can help patients improve their mental and physical health and reduce the risk of chronic diseases.

**Nutrition & Cognition:**

Another significant finding is the importance of nutrition in cognitive function and overall wellness. Research has demonstrated that certain foods and nutrients can support brain function and protect against cognitive decline (Gómez-Pinilla, 2008; Morris et al., 2015).

Over one-third of American adults are obese, with similar statistics observed worldwide. Caloric intake and diet composition significantly impact cognition and emotion, particularly during critical developmental periods; however, the neural mechanisms driving these effects remain poorly understood. A deeper understanding of the cognitive-emotional processes underlying the desire to overconsume food could inform more effective obesity prevention and treatment strategies.

This review highlights recent findings linking dietary fat intake and imbalances in omega-3 polyunsaturated fatty acids with inflammation in the developing, adult, and aging brain. It underscores how early-life dietary patterns and stress exposure can contribute to lifelong cognitive dysfunction. Early nutritional interventions, such as supplementation with essential micronutrients, show promise in mitigating these deficits.

Furthermore, acute consumption of high-fat diets primes the hippocampus to elicit an exaggerated neuroinflammatory response to mild immune challenges, leading to memory impairment. Inadequate intake of omega-3 fatty acids may also exacerbate depression by affecting endocannabinoid and inflammatory pathways in specific brain regions, triggering synaptic pruning by microglia in the hippocampus, and resulting in memory loss.

On a positive note, diets rich in polyphenol-containing fruits and vegetables can counteract age-related cognitive decline by reducing oxidative stress and inflammation. Advancing our understanding of the interplay between diet, cognition, and emotion is crucial for identifying mechanisms and developing strategies to prevent or alleviate neurological conditions associated with obesity.

The mind-gut relationship is also crucial in promoting overall wellness, as the gut microbiome has been linked to various health outcomes, including immune function, mental health, and chronic disease.

**The Role of a Nurse in Promoting Proper Health**

Nurses are critical in promoting proper nutrition and educating patients about healthy eating habits. Nurses can help patients identify and address barriers to healthy eating, such as a lack of access to healthy foods or knowledge about healthy eating habits.

Nurses can also educate and provide patients with resources about healthy eating habits. This can include information about portion control, healthy food choices, and the importance of balanced meals. Nurses can also provide information about healthy snack options and how to make healthy choices when eating out.

In addition to patient education, nurses can monitor patients' nutritional status and recommend dietary changes as needed. This may involve working with a registered dietitian to develop a customized nutrition plan for the patient. Following are some ways a nurse could be the driving force in holistic healing for their patients:

- "The nurse should assist the individual in maintaining a balanced diet."

A balanced diet is essential for good health, and nurses play an important role in helping patients understand proper nutrition and make healthy food choices.

- "The nurse should assist the individual to get adequate rest and sleep."

Adequate rest and sleep are essential for maintaining good health. Nurses must work with patients to help them establish healthy sleep habits and promote relaxation.

- "The nurse should help the individual to maintain a comfortable environment."

A comfortable environment is important for promoting healing and preventing further illness. Nurses must work to create a safe and comfortable environment for patients.

- "The nurse should attend to the patient's spiritual and cultural needs."

**Henderson** recognized the importance of addressing patients' spiritual and cultural needs in promoting overall health and well-being. Nurses must be sensitive to patients' cultural and spiritual beliefs and work to incorporate them into their care.

- "The nurse should help the individual to avoid hazards and the transmission of disease."

Preventing the spread of disease and avoiding hazards is essential for maintaining good health. Nurses must provide education and resources to help patients understand how to protect themselves from harm.

- "The nurse should help the individual to communicate effectively with others."

Effective communication is essential for maintaining social relationships and promoting overall health. Nurses must help patients develop effective communication skills and provide resources for communicating with others.

- "The nurse should help the individual to progress towards independence."

The goal of nursing care is to help patients achieve independence and self-care. Nurses must work with patients to help them develop the skills and knowledge they need to manage their health independently.

- "The nurse should help the individual to accept and adapt to the present situation."

Accepting and adapting to the present situation is important for promoting mental and emotional well-being. Nurses must provide emotional support and resources to help patients cope with their health challenges.

- "The nurse should help the individual to develop a sense of responsibility for his own health."

Taking responsibility for one's own health is essential for achieving and maintaining good health. Nurses must work with patients to help them develop a sense of responsibility for their own health and well-being.

- "The nurse should provide care in a way that is respectful of the patient's dignity."

Respect for the patient's dignity is essential for maintaining trust and promoting overall health. Nurses must provide care in a respectful and dignified manner.

- "The nurse should work collaboratively with other healthcare professionals."

Collaboration with other healthcare professionals is essential for providing comprehensive care and promoting overall health. Nurses must work with other healthcare professionals to ensure that patients receive the best possible care.

## Practicing Self-Care

Prioritizing self-care can take many forms, such as setting boundaries, engaging in regular exercise, maintaining healthy nutrition habits, and engaging in activities that promote relaxation and stress reduction. By prioritizing self-care, healthcare professionals can better manage the demands of their jobs and maintain the energy and focus needed to provide high-quality care.

**Healthy Eating:** Good nutrition is essential for maintaining physical health and reducing stress levels. Nurses can practice healthy eating habits, such as consuming a balanced diet with fruits, vegetables, lean protein, and whole grains.

As healthcare professionals, it is essential to engage in self-care techniques to prevent burnout and promote personal and professional wellness. Techniques for enhancing self-care in nursing practice include physical activities like exercise and adequate sleep, nutrition and hydration, social support, leisure activities, and hobbies. In addition, practices like meditation, prayer, and positive affirmations can be incorporated into daily routines to reduce stress, increase mindfulness, and promote a positive outlook on life.

## Strategies for Improving Nutrition in Clinical Settings

There are several strategies that nurses can use to improve nutrition in clinical settings. These strategies include:

- Conducting nutritional assessments: Nurses can use tools such as the Mini Nutritional Assessment (MNA) to assess patients' nutritional status and identify areas where dietary changes may be needed.
- Providing education and resources: Nurses can provide patients with information about healthy eating habits, such as portion control, balanced meals, and healthy snack options. Nurses can also provide resources, such as recipes and information about local farmers' markets.
- Working with a registered dietitian: Nurses can collaborate with a registered dietitian to develop customized nutrition plans for patients.
- Monitoring and documenting nutritional status: Nurses can monitor and document patients' nutritional status, including weight, body mass index (BMI), and lab values.
- Incorporating nutrition into care plans: Nurses can incorporate nutrition into care plans for patients, including setting goals for dietary changes and monitoring progress.

## Devil's Advocate

How can nurses encourage patients to adopt a plant-based diet when they may have cultural or personal beliefs that do not align with this approach?

The case of Dr. Terry Wahls is a well-known example of the healing power of nutrition. Dr. Wahls, a physician diagnosed with multiple sclerosis, was able to reverse her symptoms and achieve remission by adopting a nutrient-dense, plant-based diet.

In a case study published in the journal Integrative Cancer Therapies, a woman with breast cancer underwent a program of nutritional and lifestyle changes, as well as emotional and spiritual therapies. Despite not receiving conventional treatment, she experienced a complete remission and has been cancer-free for over 20 years. (Lipton, J. (2010).

However, nurses face challenges in advocating for policy change related to nutrition and other health issues. One major challenge is the influence of powerful industries, such as the food and beverage industry, that may resist policy changes that could impact their profits. Additionally, political gridlock and polarization can make it difficult for nurses to influence policy at the national level.

For example, if an NGO is promoting a diet that is not in line with the latest research on optimal nutrition and health outcomes, nurses must be willing to speak out and advocate for a change in policy. This may require them to challenge the consensus view within the NGO and to push for a change in direction.

Taking a stance opposing the status quo can be challenging, particularly when there is pressure to conform and maintain the current policies and practices. However, nurses have a responsibility to their patients and communities to advocate for their health needs and to push for policies that promote optimal health outcomes.

One way nursing can bring about change at a societal level is by promoting evidence-based practices in healthcare settings. As mentioned earlier, nursing education institutions can play a vital role in promoting the most current science in nutrition and other areas of healthcare. This knowledge can be disseminated to healthcare professionals through continuing education programs and other professional development opportunities. By equipping healthcare professionals with the most current evidence-based practices, nursing can help ensure patients receive the highest quality care possible.

## Conclusion

The New Nursing Theory is a comprehensive approach to healthcare that incorporates principles from various authors and concepts. It emphasizes the importance of the nurse-patient relationship, nutrition, self-care, evidence-based practice, and cultural competency. By combining these principles into practice, nurses can promote optimal health outcomes for their patients and create a more fulfilling and rewarding work environment for themselves.

Pursuing optimal nutrition is foundational to the Grand Theory, as it recognizes the importance of nutrition in maintaining health and preventing illness. A healthy diet provides the body with the necessary nutrients to function correctly and supports the body's natural healing processes.

Additionally, the theory emphasizes the importance of understanding the interconnectedness of all beings and the need for nurses to create healing environments that foster positive relationships between patients, families, and healthcare providers.

Nurses can work with patients and families to develop personalized nutrition plans that meet their needs and preferences.

This can involve education on healthy eating habits, as well as practical support with meal planning and preparation.

As we know, optimal nutrition is foundational to all wellness. Nurses can educate patients about the importance of proper nutrition and help them develop healthy eating habits. A plant-based diet, rich in fruits, vegetables, whole grains, and lean proteins, has been shown to reduce the risk of chronic diseases such as heart disease, cancer, and diabetes.

Nutrition plays a critical role in nursing practice, as it promotes health and prevents disease. Nurses play a vital role in promoting proper nutrition and educating patients about healthy eating habits. By using strategies such as nutritional assessments, patient education, and collaboration with registered dietitians, nurses can help improve nutrition in clinical settings and enhance patient outcomes.

Overall, there is a growing body of evidence demonstrating the importance of diet and lifestyle choices in the prevention and management of chronic diseases. Addressing these root causes of chronic diseases could have a significant impact on reducing healthcare costs and improving overall health outcomes. As healthcare professionals, it is important to educate patients on the importance of healthy lifestyle choices and provide them with the tools and resources they need to make positive changes in their lives.

# References

Dinan TG, Cryan JF. Gut instincts: microbiota as a key regulator of brain development, ageing and neurodegeneration. J Physiol. 2017 Jan 15;595(2):489-503. doi: 10.1113/JP273106. Epub 2016 Dec 4. PMID: 27641441; PMCID: PMC5233671.

Mörkl S, Wagner-Skacel J, Lahousen T, Lackner S, Holasek SJ, Bengesser SA, Painold A, Holl AK, Reininghaus E. The Role of Nutrition and the Gut-Brain Axis in Psychiatry: A Review of the Literature. Neuropsychobiology. 2018 Sep 17:1-9. doi: 10.1159/000492834. Epub ahead of print. PMID: 30223263.

Spencer SJ, Korosi A, Layé S, Shukitt-Hale B, Barrientos RM. Food for thought: how nutrition impacts cognition and emotion. NPJ Sci Food. 2017 Dec 6;1:7. doi: 10.1038/s41538-017-0008-y. PMID: 31304249; PMCID: PMC6550267.

# Chapter 9: Mindfulness and Nursing Practice

## A New Perspective

The New Nursing Theory celebrates and acknowledges the inevitable impact of Love and the Power of Mind and how both can orchestrate any patient's healing. The theory combines the power of the mind and the force of love, supported by quantum physics and the unified field theory. It takes the best parts of various nursing theorists to create a systematic approach to positive thinking in nursing practice. This approach, inspired by numerous case studies in science and nursing, demonstrates the effectiveness of positive thinking and its profound impact on patient outcomes, inspiring and motivating nurses to incorporate this approach into their work.

This New Theory can potentially transform nursing practice, promoting a more patient-centered, holistic approach to care. This theory proposes that love, the ubiquitous fabric of the universe, is the force for good health and healing. It also affirms that pursuing optimal nutrition is foundational to all wellness and that mindfulness practices can enhance self-care and reduce stress.

*The New Nursing Theory also promotes patient education and its critical role in promoting self-care practices that can reduce reliance on the healthcare system. In an era where chronic diseases are increasingly linked to lifestyle choices, environmental factors, and dietary habits, equipping individuals with comprehensive knowledge about their health enables them to take proactive measures to maintain well-being, prevent illness, and manage existing conditions without constant medical intervention.*

*Self-care extends beyond simply treating symptoms; it fosters a preventive mindset that integrates nutrition, mental well-being, physical activity, and holistic health practices. Studies in preventive medicine and health literacy suggest that when individuals are well-informed about the root causes of disease, they are more likely to adopt sustainable lifestyle changes that mitigate the need for frequent interactions with the healthcare system. This shift can reduce the burden on healthcare providers, lower medical costs, and ultimately minimize dependency on a system that often focuses on disease management rather than prevention.*

*Moreover, the healthcare industry operates within an economic model that benefits from sustained patient engagement. The system is largely reactive in its current structure, addressing illnesses after they manifest rather than prioritizing proactive, preventive care. By empowering individuals with education and self-care strategies, the necessity for medical intervention can be significantly minimized, allowing for a transformation in the way health and well-being are approached. This paradigm shift—from a disease-management system to a prevention-driven model—places the responsibility and power back into the hands of individuals, fostering greater autonomy, long-term wellness, and reduced reliance on institutional healthcare.*

Dr. Bruce Lipton and Dr. Gregg Braden are prominent figures whose work has significantly influenced holistic healing and patient care. Their interdisciplinary approaches—merging science, spirituality, and human potential—offer transformative insights that have implications for nursing practice and holistic healthcare. Dr. Bruce Lipton is a stem cell biologist and author best known for his work in epigenetics, particularly through his book *The Biology of Belief*. His research emphasizes how environmental factors, thoughts, emotions, and beliefs can influence gene expression, challenging the deterministic view of genetics.

The works of Dr. Bruce inspire the New Nursing Theory and emphasizes that nurses could educate patients about the power of their mindset and lifestyle choices in influencing health outcomes. This aligns with patient-centered care and the emphasis on preventive health strategies. Lipton's work validates the importance of addressing patients' emotional and psychological states, suggesting that care should focus on the physical body and emotional and mental well-being.

By recognizing the power of positive energy and self-love, nurses can create a healing environment that promotes the well-being of their patients. By incorporating holistic health practices in their own lives, such as balanced diet and nutrition, mobility, and meditation, nurses can facilitate and accelerate their patients' physical, emotional, and spiritual health improvement.

## What is Mindfulness?

Mindfulness is deliberately focusing one's attention on the present moment with an attitude of openness, curiosity, and acceptance. Rooted in ancient contemplative traditions, particularly Buddhism, mindfulness has been adapted into contemporary therapeutic and wellness practices to promote mental well-being, leading to holistic health benefits. In essence, mindfulness involves:

- **Awareness**: Maintaining conscious attention to thoughts, emotions, bodily sensations, and surrounding environment without judgment.
- **Present-Moment Focus**: Emphasizing the "here and now" rather than dwelling on the past or worrying about the future.
- **Acceptance**: Observing experiences as they unfold without trying to change or resist them.

This practice is widely recognized for its benefits in reducing stress, improving emotional regulation, enhancing focus, and fostering overall mental and physical health. It is often incorporated into interventions such as Mindfulness-Based Stress Reduction (MBSR) and Mindfulness-Based Cognitive Therapy (MBCT). Being present in the moment and aware of one's thoughts and emotions are crucial in promoting positive thought in nursing practice and healthcare as it helps both staff and patients practice self-reflection and self-awareness, cultivate a non-judgmental attitude towards oneself and others, and foster a sense of gratitude and appreciation of life as is.

The New Nursing Theory, too, believes and advocates this mind-body connection, i.e., the mind and body are interconnected and affect each other. Positive and Mindful thinking and emotions can enhance this connection and promote physical health and well-being. This theory states that thoughts and emotions impact physical health and well-being, and practices like mindfulness and positive thinking enhance the mind-body connection, improving patient outcomes in nursing care.

## Mindfulness and Orem's Self-Care Deficit Theory

In nursing practice, positive thinking, mindfulness, and self-awareness are closely related to Orem's Self-Care Deficit Theory, which highlights the importance of self-care in maintaining optimal health. According to Dorothea Orem, individuals are responsible for caring for themselves and engaging in self-care activities to prevent illness and promote well-being. The new nursing theory builds on Orem's Self-Care Deficit Theory by emphasizing the importance of positive thinking and mindfulness in promoting self-care. Studies have shown that positive thinking and mindfulness can enhance an individual's ability to engage in self-care activities and promote overall well-being (Boguszewski & Zalewska, 2020).[xxi]

One of the key concepts of Orem's theory is self-care deficit. This concept refers to situations where individuals are unable to engage in self-care activities due to various factors, including physical or mental limitations. Orem proposed that nursing interventions could assist individuals in overcoming self-care deficits. Orem's Self-Care Deficit Nursing Theory forms a key part of her broader Self-Care Framework, which focuses on the relationship between a person's capacity for self-care and the assistance required from nursing professionals.

**Core Concepts of the Self-Care Deficit Theory:**

**1. Self-Care:**

These include activities individuals initiate and perform to maintain life, health, and well-being. Self-care requisites are categorized as:

- **Universal:** Basic needs (e.g., air, water, food, elimination, rest, and social interactions).
- **Developmental:** Needs related to growth and development.
- **Health Deviation:** Needs arising from illness, injury, or treatments.

**2. Self-Care Deficit:**

It occurs when an individual cannot meet their self-care needs due to limitations caused by illness, injury, or developmental issues. This is the point where nursing intervention is required.

**3. Nursing Agency:**

It refers to the nurse's ability to assess and meet patients' self-care needs. Nurses play a role in compensating for deficits and fostering self-care ability when possible.

### 4. Nursing Systems:

Orem outlines three types of nursing systems depending on the extent of the self-care deficit:

- **Wholly Compensatory**: The nurse provides total care when the individual cannot meet self-care needs.
- **Partially Compensatory**: The nurse assists individuals who can perform some but not all self-care activities.
- **Supportive-Educative**: The nurse provides guidance or education to help individuals develop their ability to care for themselves.

## Application in Nursing Practice

Orem's Self-Care Deficit Theory is widely used in nursing practice to:

- Assess patients' needs and their ability to meet those needs.
- Plan individualized care to bridge the self-care deficit.
- Promote autonomy by enabling patients to regain their self-care capabilities when possible.

Nurses can indeed encourage patients to adopt healthy lifestyle behaviors, including a nutritious diet, regular exercise, and stress management techniques. Nurses can empower patients to take an active role in their health and wellness by educating them on the mind-body connection and the importance of positive thought and intention.[xxii]

The New Nursing Theory enhances patient-centered care by focusing on the patient's level of independence and providing appropriate support. It also helps nurses deliver effective interventions.

For instance, a study by Boguszewski and Zalewska (2020) found that mindfulness-based interventions effectively improved self-care behaviors in patients with chronic diseases. The study showed that participants who received mindfulness-based interventions reported significant improvements in their ability to engage in self-care activities, including exercise, healthy eating, and stress management.

Another study by Talaee and Najafi (2018) found that positive thinking interventions effectively improved self-care behaviors in patients with type 2 diabetes. The study showed that participants who received positive thinking interventions reported significant improvements in their ability to engage in self-care activities, including monitoring blood sugar levels, taking medication, and engaging in physical activity.[xxiii]

Overall, the connection between Orem's Self-Care Deficit Theory and the new nursing theory based on the power of the mind and the force of love is significant. The new nursing theory builds on Orem's theory by emphasizing the importance of positive thinking and mindfulness in promoting self-care behaviors. Research has shown that these concepts can enhance an individual's ability to engage in self-care activities and promote overall well-being.

## Mind-Body Connection and Healing

Recent research has provided some support for this theory of mind and love. Jean Watson's Human Caring Theory and the Carrative Principles Theory emphasize the importance of creating a healing environment that considers the whole person, including their physical, emotional, and spiritual needs. This involves focusing on human-to-human connections, compassion, empathy, and the therapeutic use of self. The power of consciousness and energy in healing and transformation aligns with Watson's theory, which recognizes that the mind-body connection is essential to health and healing. The placebo effect, for example, illustrates how the mind can influence physical health outcomes.

Studies show that placebo treatments can have a measurable effect on the brain and body, including changes in neurotransmitter activity, hormone levels, and immune function. These effects appear to be strongest when the placebo is given in a context of trust, care, and empathy. This affirms that the therapeutic relationship between the healthcare provider and patient may play a significant role in the placebo effect.

The New Nursing Theory also supports the role of belief and expectation in healing and strategies for promoting positive expectations and beliefs. One notable example is the placebo effect. Studies have shown that patients who receive a placebo treatment, which is essentially a sugar pill with no active ingredients, often report a reduction in symptoms and an improvement in their overall health. This effect, partly due to the power of positive thinking and the belief that the treatment will work, is a crucial aspect of nursing practice.

A real placebo effect is a psychobiological phenomenon occurring in the patient's brain after the administration of an inert substance or a sham physical treatment such as sham surgery, along with verbal suggestions (or any other cue) of clinical benefit (Price *et al.*, 2008). The placebo effect is when a patient's symptoms improve after receiving a treatment with no active therapeutic ingredients. It is effective in various medical conditions, including pain, depression, and anxiety. Although placebos have long been considered a nuisance in clinical research, today, they represent an active and productive field. Because of the involvement of many mechanisms, the study of the placebo effect can be viewed as a melting pot of concepts and ideas for neuroscience.

We must note that the effect that follows the administration of a placebo cannot be attributable to the inert substance alone, for saline solutions or sugar pills will never acquire therapeutic properties. Instead, the effect is because of the psychosocial context surrounding the inert substance and the patient. In this sense, the term 'placebo effect' has different meanings for clinical trialists and neurobiologists.

The placebo effect is believed to be due to the patient's expectations and beliefs about the treatment. These expectations can activate the body's natural healing processes, improving symptoms. The placebo effect has been demonstrated in numerous studies, including a meta-analysis of 130 clinical trials, which found that it accounted for an average of 30% of the improvement in symptoms.

Indeed, only a few placebo effects exist with different mechanisms and in various systems, medical conditions, and therapeutic interventions. For example, brain mechanisms of expectation, anxiety, and reward are all involved, as are a variety of learning phenomena, such as Pavlovian conditioning, cognitive, and social learning. There is also some experimental evidence of different genetic variants in placebo responsiveness.

Pain and Parkinson's disease are the most productive models for better understanding the neurobiology of the placebo effect. The placebo effect is a psychosocial context effect. The data indicates that different social stimuli, such as words and rituals of the therapeutic act, may change the chemistry and circuitry of the patient's brain. This has significant implications for nursing practice.

One approach to managing chronic pain is the use of mindfulness-based interventions. Mindfulness-based interventions, such as mindfulness meditation, are effective in reducing chronic pain and improving the quality of life in patients with chronic pain (Kabat-Zinn, 1982; Garland et al., 2012). Additionally, incorporating the principles of the Health Promotion Model (HPM) by Nola Pender can benefit this scenario. The HPM emphasizes the importance of self-efficacy, the perceived benefits of behavior change, and the impact of individual characteristics and experiences on health behavior (Pender, 1996). In Mrs. A's case, helping her develop a sense of self-efficacy and providing education on the benefits of pain management strategies can help improve her overall health outcomes.

Women with breast cancer report numerous symptoms, either from the disease itself or as a result of treatment. Psychological symptoms of stress, anxiety, depression, fear of recurrence, impaired cognitive functioning, and physical symptoms of pain, fatigue, and sleep disturbances continue after treatment ends, which negatively impact their quality of life. [xxiv]

Mindfulness-Based Stress Reduction (MBSR) is a clinical program designed to alleviate stress by training individuals in four meditative practices and emphasizing the attitudinal foundations of mindfulness. These foundations include non-judging, patience, a beginner's mind, trust, non-striving, acceptance, letting go, and compassion (Kabat-Zinn et al., 1985, 1992).

Evidence affirms that MBSR is effective in mitigating symptoms such as fatigue, mood disturbances, stress-related anxiety, depression, anger, and confusion among women diagnosed with breast cancer. While MBSR has been associated with improvements in sleep quality, it does not appear to significantly impact sleep efficiency. Furthermore, preliminary research conducted by our team has demonstrated that MBSR is beneficial for breast cancer survivors by reducing depression, anxiety, and fears of recurrence, as well as enhancing certain aspects of quality of life (Lengacher et al., 2009, 2010).

## Modulation of Anxiety by Expectations

Anxiety has been found to be reduced after placebo administration in some studies. If one expects a distressing symptom to subside shortly, anxiety tends to decrease. For example, early studies by McGlashan *et al.* (1969) and Evans (1977) investigated experimental pain in both trait and state anxiety subjects. Trait anxiety represents a personality trait and thus can be found throughout life. In contrast, state anxiety may be present in specific stressful situations and represents an adaptive and transitory response to stress. These researchers gave the subjects a placebo that they believed to be a painkiller. No correlation was found between trait anxiety and pain tolerance after placebo administration; a correlation occurred between situational anxiety and pain tolerance during the placebo session. Similar results were obtained more recently by Vase *et al.* (2005), who found decreased anxiety levels in patients with irritable bowel syndrome who received a placebo treatment.

## Holistic Approach to Patient Care

The New Nursing Theory combines the concepts of Quantum physics, the law of attraction, and the placebo effect, highlighting the relationship between mindfulness, energy, and healing. The placebo effect, for instance, is a phenomenon where a patient's belief in a treatment's effectiveness can lead to a positive health outcome, even if the treatment has no active ingredients or physiological effect.

All three concepts share a focus on the power of mindfulness and energy in healing and transformation. The placebo effect and the law of attraction both suggest that belief and positive thinking can have a tangible impact on health outcomes. At the same time, quantum physics offers a scientific framework for understanding the underlying mechanics of energy and consciousness.

Expert insights suggest that while the placebo effect and the law of attraction may not have a scientific basis, they can offer useful tools for promoting positive thinking and emotions, which can have a tangible impact on mental and physical health. By incorporating insights from all three concepts, practitioners can adopt a more holistic and compassionate approach to patient care, recognizing the complex interplay between the mind, body, and energy.

Moreover, the law of attraction and the placebo effect suggest that a positive attitude and belief in the treatment's effectiveness can have a tangible impact on health outcomes. Watson's theory emphasizes the importance of creating a healing environment that fosters positive emotions and thoughts and cultivates trust and hope.

By recognizing the interplay between consciousness, energy, and healing, practitioners can adopt a more holistic and compassionate approach to patient care that considers the whole person's needs.

## Joe Dispenza and Gregg Braden on the Superpower: PLAECBO

Throughout history up until the present, many cultures have traditionally experienced the effects of verifiable healings, along with hexes, curses, witchcraft, voodoo, and other mysterious phenomena. These effects (many of which were elicited by unscientific means) were brought about by the beliefs and lore of society. Even today, pharmaceutical companies use double-and triple-blind randomized studies to exclude the power of the mind over the body.

Joe Dispenza is an author, speaker, and chiropractor specializing in neuroscience, quantum physics, and meditation. He has written several books, including "Breaking the Habit of Being Yourself," "You Are the Placebo," and "Becoming Supernatural." In You Are the Placebo, Dr. Joe Dispenza explores the history, science, and practical applications of the placebo effect. He empowers the readers to use "the expectation of a particular outcome" to alter their internal states and external reality solely through the actions of their minds. He offers the necessary understanding to change old beliefs and perceptions into new ones. In addition, he teaches a model of personal transformation that correlates with the placebo effect without the need for any external influences).

*Braden argues that the placebo effect is a real effect and that the power of prayer could still be harnessed for healing and other purposes. Collapsing potential into physical reality is not limited to quantum physics. It has been observed in many areas of life, including medicine and psychology. For example, the placebo effect is a well-known phenomenon in which a patient's belief in a treatment can produce fundamental physiological changes in the body, even when the treatment is inactive.*

*Joe Dispenza and Gregg Braden both explore the power of the placebo effect, but from slightly different perspectives, blending neuroscience, quantum physics, and ancient wisdom. Their work highlights the mind's ability to influence physical reality, particularly in healing and transformation.*

*Dr. Joe Dispenza, a neuroscientist and researcher, delves deep into the placebo effect highlighting that belief alone can trigger physiological changes, demonstrating that the body does not distinguish between a real experience and one that is vividly imagined.*

*The brain rewires itself based on repeated thoughts, emotions, and experiences. When someone believes they are healing, their brain activates neural pathways as if the healing is already occurring. Thoughts and emotions influence gene expression. Positive expectations and emotions can activate self-healing mechanisms, while stress and negative emotions suppress immune function. Dispenza's research shows that meditation creates measurable changes in brain activity and body chemistry. Through techniques like mental rehearsal, individuals can induce physiological changes similar to those seen in people taking actual pharmaceutical drugs.*

*Dispenza argues that a placebo is not just a medical phenomenon but a superpower we can harness by consciously training the mind to generate biochemical changes in the body.*

Gregg Braden, a researcher and author, approaches the placebo effect from a quantum and energetic perspective, linking modern science with ancient spiritual wisdom. He argues that the placebo effect proves the body's ability to self-regulate and heal when consciousness and energy are aligned.

Braden demonstrates that the universe operates like a field of energy (what he calls the Divine Matrix), where thoughts and emotions directly influence reality. Studies in HeartMath Institute research show that when the heart and brain synchronize through positive emotion, the body enters an optimal healing state. Many ancient traditions (Tibetan monks, indigenous healers) use prayer, intention, and ritual to induce healing—essentially harnessing the placebo effect before science could explain it. He presents evidence of cases where tumors disappeared in real-time during focused healing sessions, showing that belief and energy shifts can override biological conditions. Braden connects the placebo effect to the idea that we exist in an intelligent, conscious universe where our thoughts, beliefs, and emotions shape physical outcomes.

*Both Dispenza and Braden suggest that a placebo is not an illusion but an untapped human potential. This biological and energetic mechanism allows the mind to heal the body and reshape reality. Their work emphasizes that by mastering belief, visualization, meditation, and heart-brain coherence, we can consciously activate the placebo effect to improve health, enhance performance, and manifest desired outcomes.*

## The Nocebo Effect

*While the Placebo Effect occurs when a person experiences a positive health outcome after receiving a treatment that has no active therapeutic ingredients, and it is believed to be due to the power of the mind to influence the body, the negative expectations arising from clinical interactions can lead to detrimental outcomes, commonly referred to as Nocebo Effects.*

*Notably, research on the Nocebo effect suggests that the mere disclosure of potential side effects may contribute to the manifestation of adverse outcomes. The nocebo response is shaped by both the content and manner in which information is conveyed to patients during clinical trials, affecting outcomes in both placebo and active treatment conditions. The Nocebo effect has a negative impact on patients' quality of life and adherence to therapy, underscoring the importance of minimizing these responses. In other words, the nocebo effect is the opposite of the placebo effect, where a person experiences negative health outcomes after being exposed to a negative expectation or belief.*

*If someone expects a treatment to be ineffective or to cause harm, they may experience negative effects even if the treatment itself is harmless or beneficial. The nocebo effect can result in a range of symptoms and conditions, including pain, nausea, dizziness, and even death in extreme cases.*

*Management of verbal communication, contextual cues associated with any treatment, and other aspects of physician-patient interactions are essential elements of good clinical practice. Potentially promising methods of reducing nocebo effects include framing information, the authorized concealment approach, educating patients about the possibility of nocebo responses, promoting optimal doctor-patient interactions, and effective management of symptoms. Future empirical research is desirable to assess various communication strategies concerning generating nocebo responses and their impact on patients' comprehension of what they need to know about adverse effects to make autonomous treatment decisions that reflect their values and preferences.*

*The placebo and nocebo effects are relevant to the new nursing theory as they highlight the significant impact of thoughts and beliefs on health outcomes. In the new nursing theory, there is an emphasis on the power of the mind-body connection and the role of positive emotions and attitudes in promoting healing and wellness.*

*In the new nursing theory, there is an emphasis on the use of mindfulness techniques, positive affirmations, and healthy lifestyle habits to promote positive beliefs and attitudes in patients. By encouraging patients to adopt a positive and optimistic outlook, healthcare providers can help promote healing and wellness and potentially even enhance the effectiveness of medical interventions. Overall, the placebo and nocebo effects serve as important reminders of the interconnectedness of the mind and body and the potential for positive change through focused attention and intentional action.*

## Mindful Self-care for Nurses

Studies have also shown that mindful self-care can have a positive impact on the mental and physical health of healthcare providers, including nurses. A study published in the Journal of

Holistic Nursing found that nurses who practiced mindfulness meditation, a technique that focuses on the present moment and cultivates a nonjudgmental awareness of thoughts and feelings, reported lower stress and anxiety levels.

Based on an analysis, the most substantial outcomes were reduced levels of emotional exhaustion (a dimension of burnout), stress, psychological distress, depression, anxiety, and occupational stress. Improvements were found in terms of mindfulness, personal accomplishment (a dimension of burnout), (occupational) self-compassion, quality of sleep, and relaxation. The systematic review results suggested that MBSR could help improve employees' psychological functioning.[xxv]

Nurses can use the placebo effect to improve patient outcomes by providing supportive care that enhances patients' expectations and beliefs about treatment. Nurses can play a critical role in fostering trust, empathy, and compassion with their patients, which may enhance the placebo effect and improve health outcomes. In addition, nurses can work to integrate mindfulness and other holistic approaches into their practice, which may help to support the mind-body connection and enhance the potential for positive health outcomes.

Studies have shown that positive communication and interactions between nurses and patients can lead to improved patient outcomes, including reduced pain, anxiety, and stress. For example, a study published in the Journal of Advanced Nursing found that nurses who used positive communication strategies with patients reported higher levels of patient satisfaction and improved patient outcomes.

The nursing theory uses examples from across cultures, such as the Chi Gung Master of Malaysia, DJ healer, Shamanism, The Hunza People of the Himalayas, and other observed examples like the placebo effect, to formulate a systematic approach to teaching the adoption of positive thought as a means of supporting the manifestation of positive life experiences as it relates to nursing practice and patient outcomes.

The placebo effect has significant implications for nursing practice, and nurses can use it to improve patient outcomes. The placebo effect is not a substitute for active therapy but can be used as a supportive measure to enhance patient expectations and beliefs about the treatment. Therapeutic communication and placebo treatments are effective ways to activate the placebo effect and improve patient outcomes. After the administration of a placebo, a clinical improvement may occur for a variety of reasons. Whereas the clinical trialist is interested in any improvement that may occur in a clinical trial, the neurobiologist is only interested in the psychosocial–psychobiological effects after administering a placebo. These include several mechanisms, such as anxiety, reward, learning, and genetics.

Therapeutic Communication Nurses can use therapeutic communication to enhance patient expectations and beliefs about the treatment. Empathic listening and positive feedback can create a supportive environment that encourages patients to believe in the treatment's effectiveness. Patients who believe in the treatment are more likely to experience the placebo effect and improve their symptoms. The mechanisms that are activated by placebos are the same as those activated by drugs, which affirms a cognitive/affective interference with drug action. Moreover, if prefrontal functioning is impaired, placebo responses are reduced or lacking, as occurs in dementia of Alzheimer's type.

Furthermore, studies have also shown that positive thinking can positively impact the mental and physical health of healthcare providers, including nurses. A study published in the Journal of Holistic Nursing found that nurses who practiced mindfulness meditation, a technique that focuses on the present moment and cultivates a nonjudgmental awareness of thoughts and feelings, reported lower stress and anxiety levels.

From a nursing perspective, the placebo effect and its potential relationship with quantum physics highlight the importance of the therapeutic relationship and the role of positive beliefs and attitudes in healthcare. Nurses can play a critical role in fostering trust, empathy, and compassion with their patients, which may enhance the placebo effect and improve health outcomes. In addition, nurses can work to integrate mindfulness and other holistic approaches into their practice, which may help to support the mind-body connection and enhance the potential for positive health outcomes.

While the relationship between the placebo effect and quantum physics remains an area of ongoing research and debate, the potential implications for healthcare and nursing are significant and warrant further exploration and consideration.

## Conclusion

In conclusion, the quantum nursing theory emphasizes the importance of understanding the interconnectedness of all things and the role of our thoughts, emotions, and beliefs in manifesting desired outcomes. By aligning ourselves with the high frequency of love and using it as a means of communication with the unified field, we can tap into its unlimited potential and create positive change in the world of nursing and beyond.

While the mechanisms behind the placebo effect are still not fully understood, it is believed that love, compassion, and care play a significant role in its effectiveness. Placebo treatments delivered with genuine warmth and empathy are more effective than those without these elements.

Lipton and Braden's work aligns with the growing emphasis on integrative medicine and holistic nursing, where the focus extends beyond symptom management to nurturing overall well-being. Their teachings inspire a future where science and spirituality complement each other, creating a comprehensive model of care. Overall, many case studies in science and nursing support the New Nursing theory proposed in this book. From the placebo effect to the power of mindfully positive communication in nursing, these studies demonstrate the tangible benefits of Mindfulness and positive thinking and its potential impact on patient outcomes.

In order to fully embrace the principles of the Quantum Nursing Theory and provide culturally sensitive care, healthcare providers must cultivate a mindfulness mindset. This involves being fully present in the moment, non-judgmentally observing thoughts and emotions, and being open to different perspectives and ways of healing. Mindfulness can be incorporated into daily practices such as meditation, deep breathing, and mindful eating. By cultivating mindfulness, healthcare providers can better understand and respect the unique cultural beliefs and practices that are integral to a patient's identity and self-care practices. This can enhance patient participation in the healing approach and ultimately lead to optimal health outcomes.

Various studies suggest that the placebo and nocebo effects can have a significant impact on cancer patients' quality of life and should be considered in cancer treatment plans. However, it is essential to note that the placebo and nocebo effects cannot cure cancer, and patients should always follow their doctor's recommended treatment plan. These examples demonstrate the power of love, compassion, and care in activating the placebo effect and promoting healing. While the exact mechanisms behind this phenomenon are not yet fully understood, it is clear that the role of love and empathy in healthcare cannot be underestimated.

It also affirms that the mind can heal the body even without actual physical intervention. Thoughts have been measured in terms of energy projections from the brain out into the physical world. The power of thought has been observed in the world of medicine and nursing in various phenomena recorded in anecdotal and formal research observations, such as the significant power of the placebo effect. Similarly, studies on the effects of meditation and mindfulness practices have found that they can lead to changes in brain structure and function and improve mental and physical health outcomes.

Whether through the lens of quantum physics, epigenetics, neuroplasticity, or the placebo effect, the convergence of empirical data and experiential accounts provides a robust foundation for the assertion that the mind has the potential to shape our external circumstances. While the precise mechanisms and limits of this influence remain the subject of ongoing investigation, the recognition of the mind's remarkable capacity to impact the world around us holds profound implications for how we understand health, healing, and the human mind.

## References

Benedetti, F., Carlino, E., & Pollo, A. (2011). How placebos change the patient's brain. Neuropsychopharmacology, 36(1), 339-354. Read Here.

Dispenza, Joe (2014). You Are The Placebo: Making Your Mind Matter. Carlsbad, California: Hay House.

Colloca, L., & Miller, F. G. (2011). The Nocebo effect and its relevance for clinical practice. Psychosomatic Medicine, 73(7), 598-603. Read Here.

Hróbjartsson, A., & Gøtzsche, P. C. (2010). Placebo interventions for all clinical conditions. Cochrane Database of System. Here.

Benedetti, F., & Amanzio, M. (2011). The placebo response: How words and rituals change the patient's brain. Patient Education and Counseling, 84(3), 413-419. doi: 10.1016/j.pec.2011.04.034

Kam-Hansen S, Jakubowski M, Kelley JM, Kirsch I, Hoaglin DC, Kaptchuk TJ, Burstein R. Altered placebo, and drug labeling changes the outcome of episodic migraine attacks. Sci Transl Med. 2014 Jan 8;6(218):218ra5. doi: 10.1126/scitranslmed.3006175. PMID: 24401940; PMCID: PMC4005597

Colloca, L., & Miller, F. G. (2011). How placebo responses are formed: a learning perspective. Philosophical Transactions of the Royal Society B: Biological Sciences, 366(1572), 1859-1869. https://doi.org/10.1098/rstb.2010.0398

Benedetti, F., Amanzio, M., & Maggi, G. (2009). Potentiation of placebo analgesia by proglumide. The Lancet, 353(9162), 1180. https://doi.org/10.1016/s0140-6736(98)07431-5

Heroux, L. (2016). A new understanding of the placebo effect: The pivotal role of the client-practitioner relationship in psychotherapy and coaching. Journal of Psychotherapy Integration, 26(2), 109-121.

# Chapter 10: HEALING ACROSS CULTURES

The New Nursing Theory emphasizes the importance of a holistic approach to healthcare that considers the interconnectedness of mind, body, and spirit and the flow of energy referred to as a 'universal life force.' The concept of a universal life force has existed in human cultures worldwide for centuries. Known by different names, such as Qi, Prana, and Mana, this force is believed to be the energy that permeates all things and sustains life. This life force can be the source of holistic healing in many cultures.

Mindfulness is a core component of the New Nursing theory, as it encourages individuals to be fully present and aware of their thoughts, emotions, and surroundings. The practice of mindfulness has been found to have numerous benefits, including reduced stress and anxiety, improved focus and attention, and increased feelings of well-being. Similarly, cultural sensitivity is a vital aspect of the New Nursing practice, as it recognizes and respects the diversity of patients and their unique beliefs and practices. Nurses can incorporate cultural sensitivity into patient care by learning about and acknowledging different cultural beliefs and practices. For example, some cultures may value traditional healing practices, such as herbal remedies or acupuncture, while others may prefer Western medicine. By recognizing and respecting these beliefs, nurses can tailor patient care to meet individual needs better and promote positive outcomes.

In this chapter, we will explore the similarities and overlaps in the beliefs surrounding the life force in different cultures and the alternate Healing methods across cultures and traditions that could enhance the transcultural application of the New Nursing Theory.

The New Nursing Theory has trans-cultural applicability, as it recognizes the interconnectedness of all beings and promotes a holistic approach to healing. By incorporating mindfulness and cultural sensitivity into patient care, nurses can provide more effective care that promotes healing across diverse cultural backgrounds. Additionally, the principles of the New Nursing Theory align with many traditional healing practices from different cultures, making it a versatile and inclusive approach to patient care.

# 1. Traditional Chinese Medicine (TCM) and Other Healing Traditions

TCM represents a comprehensive healthcare system derived from centuries of clinical practice and guided by a scientific framework of regulatory principles. TCM encompasses a distinctive set of theories and methodologies aimed at disease treatment and health promotion. These approaches include Chinese herbal medicine, dietary therapy, acupuncture, moxibustion, and non-pharmacological interventions such as Chinese bodywork or manual therapy ("Tuina") and traditional biofeedback techniques like "Qigong" and "Taijiquan."[xxvi]

Central to Chinese cultural and medical philosophy is the concept of *Qi*, regarded as the vital life force permeating all living entities. This energy is considered essential for maintaining health and serves as a fundamental tenet of TCM. Factors such as nutrition, physical activity, and emotional well-being are thought to influence *Qi*. At the same time, therapeutic practices like acupuncture, Tai Chi, and Qigong are employed to regulate and optimize its flow.

### The Chi Gung Master of Malaysia

Chi Gung (or Qigong) is an ancient Chinese practice deeply rooted in traditional Chinese medicine, philosophy, and martial arts.

While it is challenging to pinpoint a single "Master of Malaysia," Qigong is practiced widely in Malaysia and globally. It emphasizes the cultivation of "Qi," or life energy. Its approaches combine gentle physical movements, controlled breathing, meditation, and mental focus to enhance physical and emotional well-being.

Qigong is categorized into dynamic (movement-focused) and meditative (static and breath-focused) practices. The practice has shown numerous health benefits, including stress reduction, improved balance, enhanced bone density, and an immune system boost. Specific forms, like Baduanjin Qigong, have demonstrated effectiveness in preventing bone loss and reducing systolic and diastolic blood pressure, particularly in women. Studies have also highlighted its capacity to alleviate chronic pain, improve psychological well-being, and reduce anxiety and depression.

**Relevance to Nursing and Patient Care**

Incorporating Qigong into nursing practices can have transformative effects on both caregivers and patients:

- **Stress Reduction**: Nurses and patients can use Qigong to manage stress, promoting a calmer, more focused approach to caregiving and recovery.
- **Pain Management**: Chronic pain sufferers, such as those with back pain, have reported reduced pain intensity and improved mobility following Qigong interventions
- **Improved Quality of Life**: For patients with chronic conditions or undergoing rehabilitation, Qigong offers a holistic approach that integrates physical movement with emotional healing, supporting a quicker recovery.
- **Empathy and Compassion Training**: By practicing mindfulness through Qigong, nurses can deepen their ability to provide empathetic care

By integrating Qigong into clinical settings, healthcare providers can offer an evidence-based, non-invasive, and accessible way to complement conventional treatments, fostering holistic healing.

## 2. Hinduism - Prana

In Hinduism, Prana is the life force that permeates all things and is responsible for consciousness and vitality. It is believed to be connected to the breath, and practices such as Pranayama aim to control and enhance this energy. Prana is also seen as the subtle energy that governs the chakras, or energy centers, in the body.

The concept of *Prana*—a term that translates literally to "life"—carries profound and expansive significance in Vedic and Ayurvedic traditions. Far beyond its literal interpretation, *Prana* encompasses the multifaceted elements that sustain and regulate life, including breath, vitality, spirit, and the processes of respiration and inhalation. Ayurvedic literature richly elaborates on the importance of *Prana*, highlighting it as a critical force that underpins physical and spiritual well-being.

In Ayurvedic texts, *Prana* is frequently equated with *Vayu* (air or vital energy) and described as both a type of *Vayu* and a subtle, vital element referred to as "subtle *Prana*." This life force is said to be centered in the *nabhi* (navel), which, according to the sage Rishi Parashar, is the first organ to develop in the fetus. The *nabhi* serves as the hub for *Prana* and bodily *Ushma* (heat), emphasizing its foundational role in sustaining life. The interplay between *Agni* (digestive fire) and *Prana* further illustrates this vitality, with *Prana* being regarded as a precursor to metabolic and physiological processes.

Ayurvedic classics such as the *Charaka Samhita* introduce the concept of "Dasa Pranayatana," or the ten seats of life, which identify the vital loci within the body where *Prana* resides.

Similarly, Acharya Sushruta, in the *Sushruta Samhita*, elaborates on the twelve forms of *Prana*, encompassing elements such as *Agni*, *Soma* (the moon's essence), *Vayu*, and the mental faculties of *Satwa*, *Raja*, and *Tama*. Together with the five sensory organs (Indriyas) and the individual soul (Bhutatma), these collectively define the human essence. Additionally, *Ojas*, the vital essence of all body tissues (*Dhatus*), is intrinsically linked to *Prana*, serving as its reservoir and manifestation within the body.

## Spanda

Ancient sages from the lineage of Shaiva Tantra recognized that a pulsing energy, which they called Spanda, is at the heart of all phenomena. They also believed that these vibrating pulses of conscious energy have an emotional flavor, which is bliss. Shaiva Tantra is a spiritual and philosophical tradition that emerged in ancient India. It is believed that this 'pulse' that is at the heart of everything is considered the form that Shakti, the feminine aspect of God, takes when she whirls out of the enduring, timeless field of consciousness, Shiva (the masculine aspect of God), and dances it into different temporary structures and creations; atoms, stars, planets, life, us.

The Universe is, therefore, essentially an ecstatic dance of the goddess. If we can unravel the temporal form of stuff, the fiber at its heart is a pulse of quivering love. 'Spanda is the pulsation of the ecstasy of Divine Consciousness.'

### Relevance to Nursing Practice

Understanding the concept of Prana offers significant insights into holistic care in nursing practice, particularly in promoting physical, emotional, and spiritual well-being. As a foundational principle in Ayurveda, *Prana* emphasizes the interconnectedness of bodily functions, mental health, and environmental influences. This perspective aligns with modern nursing's emphasis on patient-centered care, which integrates physical health with emotional and psychological support.

The focus on the navel (*nabhi*) as the center of vitality highlights the importance of core stability and central regulation in maintaining health; a concept echoed in modern practices such as neonatal care and critical care nursing. Similarly, the association between *Prana* and *Ojas* underscores the importance of nourishing interventions, emphasizing adequate nutrition and restorative practices to enhance resilience and immunity.

Moreover, the Ayurvedic view of *Prana* as a subtle and vital force aligns with nursing practices that involve mindfulness, breathwork, and relaxation techniques, which have proven benefits in managing stress, improving respiratory health, and fostering holistic healing. By integrating these principles, nurses can enhance patient outcomes through interventions that respect and support the body's natural energies, fostering a balance between health's physiological, emotional, and spiritual dimensions.

# 3. Hawaiian Culture – Mana – The Life Force of Healing

In Hawaiian culture, Mana is the life force that gives power and vitality to all things. It is believed to be present in all living and nonliving things, including rocks, trees, and animals. Mana is seen as a vital force that can be transferred between people and objects and can be harnessed through practices such as Hula dancing.

In Hawaiian culture, the concept of *Mana* represents a deeply spiritual and powerful force, central to the worldview of many Polynesian traditions. *Mana* is often described as a form of divine or supernatural power that permeates the universe, existing within people, objects, and nature. It is both a universal energy and a personal essence, deeply intertwined with an individual's actions, status, and connection to the sacred.

### Key Aspects of Mana in Hawaiian Culture:

1. **Source and Presence**:

    - *Mana* is believed to originate from divine sources, often associated with the gods (*akua*) and ancestral spirits (*aumakua*). It exists everywhere and in everything—land (*'āina*), ocean (*kai*), mountains (*mauna*), and living beings.

    - Every person is born with a degree of *mana*, which can be cultivated, enhanced, or diminished through actions and choices.

2. **Acquisition and Cultivation**:

    - *Mana* is not static; it can grow through righteous deeds, adherence to cultural practices, and spiritual discipline. Conversely, wrongdoing, disrespect, or imbalance in relationships with others and the environment can be lost or diminished.

    - Leaders and chiefs (*ali'i*) were often considered to possess high levels of *mana*, which legitimized their authority and guided their governance.

3. **Manifestations in Nature and Ritual**:

    - Natural phenomena such as storms, volcanic eruptions, or abundant harvests were often interpreted as manifestations of *mana*. Sacred sites (*heiau*) and natural features like certain trees, stones, or waterfalls were believed to be imbued with concentrated *mana*.

- o Rituals, prayers, and offerings were integral in acknowledging and honoring *mana*, ensuring harmony and balance within the community and with the spiritual world.

4. **Interconnectedness and Balance**:

    - o Hawaiian culture emphasizes the interconnectedness of all life, and *mana* is a unifying force that reflects this relationship. It fosters respect for nature, ancestors, and community.

    - o Maintaining balance (*pono*) is key. Actions that disrupt harmony or violate sacred principles (*kapu*) can negatively impact an individual's or community's *mana*.

**Relevance of Mana in Contemporary Contexts:**

Even today, the concept of *mana* influences Hawaiian identity, cultural practices, and environmental stewardship. It inspires respect for heritage, promotes sustainable practices, and fosters a deep connection with the land and its resources. The recognition of *mana* in people also underlines the importance of dignity, personal integrity, and respect in relationships.

**Broader Implications:**

The idea of *mana* offers a framework for understanding power and spirituality not as dominance but as responsibility, balance, and alignment with universal forces. This perspective encourages mindfulness in interacting with others and the environment, emphasizing harmony and collective well-being.

The Hawaiian concept of *Mana*—a spiritual energy that exists in people, objects, and nature—has profound relevance to the practice of nursing, particularly in holistic, patient-centered, and culturally sensitive care. *Mana* offers insights into the interconnectedness of health, spirituality, and well-being, which align closely with modern nursing principles.

**Relevance of *Mana* to Nursing Practice**

- **Holistic Approach to Health**:
    - In Hawaiian culture, *Mana* emphasizes the balance of physical, emotional, and spiritual energies. Similarly, nursing care encompasses not only physical health but also mental and emotional well-being.
    - Nurses can integrate this understanding by acknowledging the spiritual or cultural beliefs of patients, fostering a deeper connection between care providers and patients.

- **Empowerment and Patient Advocacy**:
    - *Mana* is believed to grow through positive actions and respect, paralleling the nursing role in empowering patients. Nurses act as advocates, helping patients build resilience and regain control over their health, much like cultivating *Mana* in a person.
    - By recognizing the unique strengths and energies of each patient, nurses can support them in their healing journey, ensuring their dignity and autonomy are respected.

- **Cultural Sensitivity and Respect**:
  - *Mana* calls for reverence toward individuals, their environment, and their traditions. Nurses can apply this by practicing cultural competence, understanding patients' values, and tailoring care to respect their beliefs and preferences.
  - For example, in multicultural healthcare settings, acknowledging *Mana* or equivalent spiritual concepts can enhance trust and communication with Native Hawaiian patients and other Indigenous communities.

- **Environmental and Community Health**:
  - *Mana* reflects the interconnectedness of people and their environment, highlighting the importance of maintaining balance. This resonates with public health nursing, which focuses on community well-being and environmental health.
  - Nurses can advocate for sustainable practices in healthcare and community wellness initiatives, promoting health in harmony with the environment.

- **Healing and Sacred Space**:
  - *Mana* emphasizes creating and preserving sacred spaces. In nursing, this translates to creating a healing environment—clean, calm, and supportive—for patients and families.
  - Practices such as mindfulness, therapeutic communication, and a respectful atmosphere honor the patient's Mana and contribute to their healing.

- **Balance and Self-Care for Nurses**:
    - The concept of *Mana* also underscores the need for balance and self-care among caregivers. As holders of healing energy, nurses must replenish their own *Mana* through self-care practices, mindfulness, and seeking support from their communities.
    - This not only sustains their ability to provide care but also models holistic well-being for their patients.

**Application in Nursing Practice**

Incorporating the principles of *Mana* into nursing care could involve:

- **Spiritual Assessment**: Including questions about cultural and spiritual beliefs in patient assessments to better understand their worldview and needs.

- **Cultural Competence Training**: Educating nurses on Hawaiian and other Indigenous traditions to enhance their ability to deliver culturally sensitive care.

- **Holistic Interventions**: Utilizing complementary therapies, such as mindfulness, nature-based activities, or traditional healing practices, to align with the patient's belief systems.

- **Community Engagement**: Collaborating with Indigenous leaders and organizations to integrate cultural values like *Mana* into public health programs and policies.

The concept of *Mana* enriches nursing by emphasizing balance, respect, and interconnectedness. By integrating these principles, nurses can enhance patient care, foster holistic healing, and build culturally sensitive practices that honor the spiritual dimensions of health and well-being.

## 4. Native American Culture - Spirit

In Native American cultures, the concept of spirit is closely tied to the life force. It is believed that all things possess a spirit, which connects them to the natural world and the Creator. Practices such as sweat lodges and vision quests aim to connect individuals with their own spirits and the spirits of the world around them. Another example can be found in the Native American tradition, which speaks of the concept of Manitou. Manitou is the spiritual energy that is believed to exist in all things and is said to be responsible for maintaining balance and harmony in the natural world.

## Shamanism and Its Relevance to Nursing Practice

Shamanism is one of the oldest spiritual and healing traditions found in diverse cultures worldwide. It is rooted in the belief that shamans—spiritual intermediaries—can access altered states of consciousness to connect with spiritual realms, seeking guidance or healing for individuals or communities. Core practices include:

1. **Journeying**: Entering a trance state to seek wisdom or healing.
2. **Energy Healing**: Removing negative energies or restoring energetic balance.
3. **Nature Connection**: Engaging with natural elements and their spiritual aspects.
4. **Rituals and Symbols**: Using tools like drumming, chanting, or sacred objects to facilitate transformation.

Shamanism emphasizes holistic healing, addressing not just physical ailments but also emotional, spiritual, and community-related imbalances.

## Relevance to Nursing Practice

Incorporating shamanic principles into nursing can enhance holistic care approaches by focusing on the interconnectedness of mind, body, and spirit. While not directly integrating traditional shamanic rituals, nurses can adopt their philosophies and practices to complement modern medicine:

### 1. Holistic Patient Care

Shamanism highlights the importance of treating patients as whole beings rather than focusing solely on symptoms. Nurses can integrate this by considering patients' emotional, psychological, and spiritual needs during care planning.

### 2. Mindfulness and Presence

Like shamanic practices, mindfulness encourages being present and fully engaged, which can enhance the therapeutic relationship between nurses and patients. This presence allows patients to feel heard and supported.

### 3. Energy Healing and Stress Reduction

Practices inspired by shamanism, such as reiki or visualization techniques, can reduce patient stress and promote relaxation. These methods align with complementary therapies used in nursing.

### 4. Cultural Competency

Understanding shamanic traditions can help nurses respect and incorporate patients' cultural and spiritual beliefs into care, fostering trust and adherence to treatment plans.

5. **Burnout Prevention**

Shamanic self-care practices, such as grounding exercises, connection with nature, and rituals for releasing emotional burdens, can help nurses manage workplace stress and prevent burnout.

## Challenges and Ethical Considerations

Integrating shamanic practices into nursing requires sensitivity to cultural authenticity and patient preferences. Nurses must also ensure complementary practices align with evidence-based care and professional ethics.

### Evidence-Based Applications

Shamanic-inspired practices, such as guided imagery, drumming for stress reduction, and energy work, have been studied for their positive effects on pain management, emotional well-being, and patient satisfaction in various healthcare settings. For example, studies indicate that drumming can induce relaxation, lower blood pressure, and alleviate chronic pain.

With shamanic insights from modern nursing frameworks, healthcare providers can create a compassionate, integrative approach that supports healing on all levels. For further exploration, texts like *Shamanism in Clinical Practice* provide detailed insights into these applications.

## Chi Kung Master DJ Healer and His Approach to Healing through Positive Thought

Chi Kung Master DJ Healer is known for incorporating the principles of Taoist energy practices, including harnessing and channeling positive thought and energy to promote physical and emotional healing. His approach aligns with ancient Chi Kung

(Qigong) techniques, emphasizing energy circulation, mindfulness, and harmony between the body, mind, and spirit.

**Core Elements of Master DJ's Healing Approach:**

- **Energy Balancing through Positive Thought**:
  Central to his practice is the belief that positive emotions and thoughts can influence energy flow, enabling the body to heal itself. This aligns with Taoist principles of balancing "Chi" (life energy) to prevent blockages that cause emotional or physical ailments.
- **Six Healing Sounds Technique**:
  Master DJ emphasizes the use of sound vibrations linked to specific organs. For example, specific sounds and visualizations target negative emotions like fear, anger, or sadness stored in organs such as the liver or lungs, replacing them with positive counterparts like kindness, courage, and love. This practice encourages mindfulness and self-awareness, aiding stress relief and emotional health.
- **The Microcosmic Orbit**:
  A foundational practice in Taoist healing involves directing energy through a loop along the spine and front of the body, known as the Microcosmic Orbit. This practice enhances vitality and supports emotional and physical balance.
- **Protective and Grounding Practices**:
  Techniques like the Iron Shirt Chi Kung focus on creating energetic resilience, protecting healers from absorbing negative energies during patient interactions, and maintaining personal equilibrium.

## Application to Nursing and Patient Care:

1. **Emotional Support**: Nurses can adapt these methods to manage their stress and support patients in emotional regulation. For example, teaching patients to visualize positive emotions can enhance their sense of well-being.
2. **Holistic Healing**: By integrating mindfulness and energy awareness techniques, caregivers can address not just the physical but also the emotional and spiritual aspects of healing, promoting a more comprehensive recovery.
3. **Stress Management**: The grounding practices in Chi Kung can help nurses manage the emotional demands of their profession, reducing burnout and improving patient interactions.
4. **Patient Empowerment**: Sharing simple energy-balancing techniques with patients can give them the tools to actively participate in their healing journey, fostering independence and resilience.

Master DJ's teachings bridge ancient wisdom with modern applications, providing valuable insights for enhancing holistic healthcare practices. For more about similar practices, we can also see the works of Taoist practitioners like Mantak Chia, who share related philosophies in accessible ways (Positive et al. Foundation).

In conclusion, Chi Gung is an ancient Chinese practice that involves using breath and movement to cultivate and direct the body's energy, or chi. It has been practiced for thousands of years and is believed to have many physical and mental health benefits. One of the most remarkable aspects of Chi Gung is its ability to harness and direct the body's energy in powerful ways. This has been demonstrated by Chi Gung masters like "DJ" from Malaysia, who has gained attention for his ability to ignite paper with focused Chi.

The technique used by "DJ" is known as "external energy manifestation," which involves channeling energy from the body's core to the hands and then directing it outward in a focused beam. This energy can be intense enough to light paper or even start a fire.

While this ability may seem extraordinary, it is a testament to the power of the human body and its ability to harness and direct energy. Chi Gung is a practice that anyone can learn and cultivate, and its benefits can extend beyond just physical health to mental and emotional well-being.

Incorporating Chi Gung practices into daily life can increase energy, improve focus and concentration, reduce stress and anxiety, and create a greater sense of calm and balance. By learning to harness and direct our body's energy, we can tap into our full potential and live more fulfilling lives.

## Some More Healing Practices Across Cultures

1. In some Native American cultures, healing practices often incorporate traditional plants and herbs, such as sage and cedar, for purification and spiritual cleansing. Practitioners may also use ritual drumming and chanting to promote relaxation and spiritual connection (Baldwin, 2018).
2. In Chinese culture, acupuncture and traditional herbal medicine are commonly used to promote physical and emotional balance. Practices such as tai chi and qigong are also used to enhance the mind-body connection and promote overall well-being (Zhang, 2019).
3. In Hindu culture, Ayurvedic medicine promotes balance and harmony between the mind, body, and spirit. This system of medicine incorporates practices such as yoga, meditation, and herbal remedies to support overall health and well-being (Sharma, 2020).

4. In African cultures, the life force is often referred to as "Ase" or "Ashé," which represents the vital energy that flows through all things. Ase is believed to be the force that connects all living things and is necessary for balance and harmony in life. It is closely tied to the concept of destiny and is believed to be present in all things. Ashe is also seen as a force that can be channeled through ritual and prayer to bring about positive change.
5. In the ancient Greek culture, the life force was known as "Pneuma," which represented the vital breath that sustained life. Pneuma was believed to be the source of all creation and was associated with the soul and the spirit.
6. The Jewish culture also has a concept of the life force known as "Ruach," representing the breath of life that sustains all living things. It is believed that by nurturing and cultivating Ruach, humans can connect with the divine and achieve spiritual fulfillment.
7. In the Islamic culture, the life force is known as "Ruh," representing the breath of life that sustains all living things. It is believed that by cultivating Ruh, humans can connect with the divine and achieve spiritual enlightenment.

In summary, many cultures across the globe have a concept of the life force, representing the vital energy that flows through all living things. Despite different names and interpretations, the underlying belief is consistent – that everything in the universe is connected.

# Importance of Cultural Sensitivity in Healthcare and Healing

To effectively apply alternative healing practices in a transcultural context, it is essential to acknowledge and respect the diversity of cultural beliefs and practices. Healthcare providers must recognize that different cultures may have unique approaches to self-care and healing and should work to incorporate these perspectives into their treatment plans. For example, in some cultures, meditation may be seen as a religious practice, while in others, it may be viewed as a secular technique for stress reduction. Healthcare providers can create a more supportive and inclusive healing environment by understanding and respecting these cultural differences.

One example of a cultural approach to mindfulness is the practice of yoga in India. Yoga is a physical and spiritual practice used for centuries to promote physical, mental, and spiritual health. In the United States, mindfulness-based stress reduction (MBSR) has been adapted from Buddhist meditation practices and has become a popular secular approach to mindfulness. These examples illustrate a variety of healing. Indeed, here are five more cultural examples:

In some indigenous cultures in the Americas, balance and harmony with nature are important for overall health and well-being. Practices such as herbal medicine, sweat lodges, and smudging ceremonies maintain this balance and promote healing (Baker, 2015; Duran, 2006).

In traditional Chinese culture, the concept of Qi (pronounced "chee") is believed to be a vital energy that flows through the body. Practices such as acupuncture and Tai Chi regulate and balance Qi's flow for physical and emotional health (Lee, Ernst, & Kok, 2010; Zhang, 2005).

In Hinduism, Ayurveda is a traditional system of medicine that emphasizes the interconnectedness of the mind, body, and spirit. Practices such as yoga, meditation, and herbal remedies are used to promote balance and harmony for optimal health (Tirtha, 2018; Singh & Rastogi, 2014).

In many African cultures, traditional healers play an important role in healthcare, using a combination of spiritual, herbal, and physical therapies to promote healing and wellbeing (Mbiti, 1991; Kofi-Tsekpo, 2013).

In Japanese culture, the concept of "wa" or harmony is important for health and wellbeing. Practices such as forest bathing (Shinrin-yoku), meditation, and tea ceremonies are used to promote relaxation and inner peace (Ohtsuka, Yabunaka, & Takayama, 2020; Sakairi, 2016).

Nurses can teach patients these techniques and practices in a variety of settings, such as in a one-on-one session or in a group class. Nurses need to have a solid understanding and personal practice of mindfulness before teaching it to patients. This can be achieved through participating in mindfulness-based programs such as Mindfulness-Based Stress Reduction (MBSR) or Mindfulness-Based Cognitive Therapy (MBCT), which have been shown to be effective in reducing stress, anxiety, and depression (Hoge et al., 2013; Wong et al., 2016). Nurses can also incorporate mindfulness into their daily routine, such as taking a few moments to focus on their breath before entering a patient's room or using mindfulness techniques to manage their own stress levels.

## Conclusion

Everything in the universe comprises energy, or life force, including human beings and their thoughts and emotions. The energy of thoughts and emotions can significantly impact an individual's physical and mental health. Energy is always moving and evolving, and nursing practice should acknowledge and work with this dynamic energy. The New Nursing Theory proposed in this book acknowledges that the human body can self-heal, and nursing interventions should aim to facilitate and enhance this innate healing ability. The power of intention and visualization can significantly impact an individual's health outcomes and healing process.

The New Nursing theory is a holistic approach to healthcare that incorporates principles of quantum physics, energy medicine, and spiritual practices. It recognizes the interconnectedness of all things and the role of consciousness in shaping reality. By utilizing techniques to manipulate one's own energy field, individuals can influence their physical and emotional states, leading to improved health and well-being. The theory offers a new paradigm for healthcare that prioritizes a personalized and integrative approach to healing.

The examples shared in this chapter are just a few of the many cultural beliefs in a universal life force or energy that exists within all things. They demonstrate the consistency and overlap of these beliefs across different cultures and periods and provide further evidence for the existence of a universal life force. Practicing mindfulness and meditation can help individuals tap into their inner energy and enhance their physical and mental well-being. The interconnectedness of all things in the universe should be recognized and integrated into nursing practice. Nursing practice should be focused on empowering individuals to take an active role in their own healing process, utilizing the principles of quantum physics and energy.

By embracing this perspective, nurses can help to create a healing environment that promotes wellness and wholeness for their patients, as well as for themselves and their colleagues. The New nursing theory represents an exciting and innovative approach to healthcare that has the potential to revolutionize the way we think about and deliver care to patients. Research has shown that practices such as meditation, prayer, and positive affirmations can significantly improve physical health outcomes, including reductions in pain, inflammation, and other symptoms of illness.

The New Nursing theory is a framework that seeks to integrate the principles of quantum physics and other sciences with nursing practice. This theory proposes that we are energetic beings in an energy-based universe and that our thoughts and emotions can influence the energetic field around us, which in turn can affect our health and wellbeing.

# References

Baldwin, J. (2018). Traditional Native American Healing. Journal of the American Academy of Psychiatry and the Law, 46(3), 397-404.

Sharma, H. (2020). Ayurvedic medicine. Journal of Ayurveda and Integrative Medicine, 11(1), 1-2.

Zhang, A. L. (2019). Acupuncture and Chinese herbal medicine: An overview of the clinical evidence. Australian Journal of Acupuncture and Chinese Medicine, 14(1), 7-14.

Luk, S. W. (2018). Chi Gung: Chinese healing, energy and natural magic. Tuttle Publishing.

Matos LC, Machado JP, Monteiro FJ, Greten HJ. Understanding Traditional Chinese Medicine Therapeutics: An Overview of the Basics and Clinical Applications. Healthcare (Basel). 2021 Mar 1;9(3):257. doi: 10.3390/healthcare9030257. PMID: 33804485; PMCID: PMC8000828.

Pandey, Smriti & Garg, Prof. (2021). THE CONCEPT OF PRANA IN AYURVEDA. World Journal of Pharmaceutical Research. 10. 493-499. 10.20959/wjpr202114-22310.

Mānoa Heritage Center. "What Is Mana?" Accessed December 9, 2024.
https://www.manoaheritagecenter.org/moolelo/kuka%CA%BBo%CA%BBo-heiau/what-is-mana/

Quantum Healing Pathways. "Mana in Hawaiian Culture and Healing Practices." Accessed December 9, 2024. https://quantumhealingpathways.com/understanding-mana/

Mālama Hawai'i. "Mana: The Spiritual Energy of Hawaiian Culture." Accessed December 9, 2024. https://www.malamahawaii.org/cultural-awareness/mana-spiritual-energy

Willetts, R. F. (1987). African Mythology. New York: Peter Bedrick Books.

# Conclusion

This book serves as a transformative guide to integrating the profound forces of the mind and love into nursing practice. By embracing a conscious and systematic approach to mindful thinking, nurses can elevate patient care, enhance their own well-being, and contribute to the evolution of the nursing profession.

This approach challenges the traditional, technology-driven focus on disease management, advocating instead for a holistic model that weaves together the art of compassionate care and the science of healing. When nurses anchor their consciousness in love and intentionality, they cultivate healing environments that honor the entirety of the human experience, fostering not only physical recovery but also emotional and spiritual renewal.

Here, love is not merely an emotion; it is a powerful, life-affirming force that enables nurses to connect deeply with their patients, offering comfort, hope, and a profound sense of belonging. This transcendent love becomes the foundation of healing, elevating nursing from a profession to a calling—one that not only mends the body but also nourishes the soul.

While the integration of positive thinking into healthcare is often associated with self-help philosophy, a growing body of scientific evidence confirms its tangible impact on well-being. Research has shown that positive thinking reshapes neural pathways, enhances resilience, and significantly improves both physical and mental health outcomes. By harnessing this power, nurses can become catalysts for profound healing, ensuring that their care extends beyond treatment—toward transformation.

Across spiritual and philosophical traditions, God is often described as omniscient (all-knowing), omnipotent (all-powerful), and omnipresent (ever-present). These attributes align with the concept of Universal Intelligence—an infinite, organizing force that governs the cosmos with precision, wisdom, and purpose. This intelligence is evident in the laws of physics, the intricate patterns of nature, and the profound interconnection of all living beings. However, intelligence alone does not sustain existence—it must be infused with love. Love is the animating force that gives meaning to intelligence, transforming mere order into harmony and structure into purpose.

If Universal Intelligence is the architect of existence, Universal Love is its foundation. Intelligence designs the universe, but love breathes life into it, binding all creation in an intricate dance of unity, balance, and purpose. Love is not just an emotion but a fundamental force—an energy that nurtures, sustains, and connects all things.

Universal Intelligence and Love are not separate; they are two aspects of the same divine reality. Intelligence provides the blueprint, and love fills it with life. This synergy is reflected in the human experience—when knowledge is applied with love, it becomes wisdom; when systems operate with love, they foster harmony.

Thus, existence itself is an expression of both intelligence and love. The galaxies move in perfect order, yet stars are born and nurtured in cosmic nurseries. The body heals itself with intricate biological precision, yet it thrives when nurtured with care. Life is not a mere mechanism; it is a masterpiece of love and wisdom interwoven.

To live in alignment with this truth is to recognize that knowledge without love is cold calculation, and love without wisdom is ungrounded idealism. True healing, whether in the body, the mind, or the soul, happens at the intersection of both—when intelligence and love work together as the fundamental forces of existence.

The emergence of quantum computing represents a fundamental shift in how we process information, mirroring the deeper intelligence woven into the fabric of the universe. Unlike classical computing, which operates on binary logic (0s and 1s), quantum computing harnesses the principles of superposition and entanglement, allowing for an exponentially higher level of interconnected computation. This interconnectedness reflects the essence of Universal Intelligence, where reality is not linear but multidimensional, operating through complex relationships rather than isolated fragments.

At its core, quantum mechanics suggests that consciousness and observation play a role in shaping reality. In the same way, Universal Intelligence is a vast field of interconnected wisdom, guiding the structure of existence at both the seen and unseen levels. The more we explore quantum computing, the more we see parallels to how intelligence operates beyond human cognition—through simultaneous possibilities, vast interconnections, and the collapse of infinite potentials into a singular reality.

Just as quantum computing transcends classical limitations, quantum healing transcends conventional medicine, recognizing that healing occurs beyond just the physical level. Quantum physics has demonstrated that particles respond to observation and intention—suggesting that consciousness itself has the power to shape matter. This aligns with the ancient spiritual understanding that love is not merely an emotion, but a vibrational force that influences reality at the deepest levels.

The New Nursing Theory proves that in the healing process, love operates as an energetic frequency that brings coherence and harmony. Studies in neuroscience and heart-brain coherence have shown that states of love, gratitude, and compassion create measurable shifts in the body—lowering stress hormones, enhancing immune response, and even altering gene expression. This supports the idea that love, much like quantum entanglement, creates an unseen yet profound connection between all things.

Just as two entangled particles affect each other instantaneously regardless of distance, healing energy, love, and intention can transcend physical space. This may explain the efficacy of prayer, energy healing, and distant healing practices. Quantum systems exist in multiple states until observed, mirroring the power of belief and intention in healing. When we hold a healing-focused consciousness, we align ourselves with a reality where healing is possible. Just as quantum coherence enables particles to function in a synchronized state, love brings the body, mind, and soul into a harmonious, healing rhythm.

Quantum computing is teaching us that reality is not deterministic but fluid, shaped by interaction and observation. Similarly, healing is not just a mechanical process but a deeply interconnected phenomenon influenced by intention, belief, and love. If Universal Intelligence is the mind of creation, then Love is its heartbeat—guiding the universe toward greater coherence, unity, and balance. In embracing both, we unlock a new paradigm of healing, where technology, consciousness, and compassion converge to redefine what is possible.

Healing extends beyond the physical body and into the realms of consciousness, intention, and human connection. Jean Watson's Theory of Human Caring provides a holistic approach to health, emphasizing the power of love, compassion, and presence as fundamental healing forces. This paper explores Watson's carative principles in relation to emerging research on the subconscious mind, quantum consciousness, and energy-based healing, demonstrating how intentional thought, belief, and emotional states influence well-being. By integrating Watson's principles with the Law of Assumption, quantum theories, and mind-body medicine, this paper presents a framework where healing is understood as a function of both science and consciousness.

Traditional medical models focus on curative approaches that target disease at the physiological level. However, Watson's carative approach emphasizes a holistic, human-centered model of care, recognizing that healing involves not just the body but also the mind, emotions, and spirit. Her ten Carative Factors, later refined into the Clinical Caritas Processes, stress the role of love, intention, and deep presence in fostering healing.

This perspective aligns with research in psychoneuroimmunology, the placebo effect, and quantum consciousness, all of which suggest that the observer (mind and consciousness) plays an active role in shaping reality. Furthermore, this model connects with Neville Goddard's Law of Assumption, which posits that deeply held beliefs and assumptions manifest into physical reality.

Train nurses to use mindfulness and visualization techniques to set positive intentions before patient interaction. Before starting a shift, nurses could take 2–3 minutes to visualize themselves providing compassionate, effective care, setting a positive tone for the day. Provide patients with tools like guided imagery recordings, affirmation cards, or visualization scripts tailored to their conditions. A heart failure patient could visualize their heart growing stronger with every beat while repeating, "My heart is healthy and powerful."

Encourage nurses to use positive, reassuring language that reinforces the patient's ability to heal. Instead of saying, "This might be difficult," a nurse could say, "You are strong, and I believe in your ability to get through this."

Integrate cultural practices that align with the patient's beliefs into care delivery, amplifying the power of intention by respecting their worldview. For a patient who believes in prayer, nurses can encourage prayer rituals while maintaining a positive presence.

One of Watson's key principles is that human connection and emotional presence are not just psychological comforts but active healing forces. This notion resonates with the idea that the subconscious mind serves as a gateway to the divine matrix, the interconnected energetic field that underlies all existence.

When the mind is still and free from external distractions—as in meditation, prayer, or deep contemplation—it becomes more receptive to healing influences. Neuroscientific research demonstrates that meditative states reduce stress hormones, enhance immune function, and promote neuroplasticity, reinforcing Watson's principle that a calm and loving environment fosters healing.

Watson's emphasis on authentic presence, loving-kindness, and transpersonal caring aligns with quantum theories that suggest consciousness is an active participant in reality. At the core of Watson's philosophy is the belief that love is the essence of healing. This idea aligns with the view that love, consciousness, and the divine matrix are interconnected, forming the foundation of reality. If consciousness shapes experience, then love—its most cohesive and potent expression—is the force that binds and heals.

This principle also connects with Neville Goddard's Law of Assumption, which posits that by assuming a state of love, wholeness, and well-being, one can manifest those qualities in their reality. From a quantum perspective, aligning one's thoughts, emotions, and beliefs with a desired state creates a vibrational match with the unified field, reinforcing Watson's assertion that healing occurs in the presence of positive intention and deep human connection.

Jean Watson's carative principles offer a transformative model of care that extends beyond the physical realm into the dimensions of consciousness, energy, and intentional healing. By integrating her work with insights from quantum physics, the subconscious mind, and the Law of Assumption, a new paradigm of health emerges—one that acknowledges the profound influence of belief, emotion, and love in shaping human well-being. Healing is not merely a biological process but a dynamic interplay of consciousness, energy, and connection, reinforcing the idea that the mind is a powerful force in shaping health and reality.

In conclusion, the concept of life force energy has been recognized across many cultures and spiritual traditions. While modern science has been slow to acknowledge its existence, recent quantum physics discoveries demonstrate a scientific basis for this phenomenon. From a spiritual and metaphysical perspective, the life force energy is the essence of the divine that animates all living things, connecting us to the larger universe. By understanding and harnessing this energy, we can promote physical, emotional, and spiritual well-being and deepen our connection to the fundamental unity of all things.

The New Nursing Theory of Love recognizes that every individual is not merely a biological entity but an interconnected field of energy and consciousness, where health is the result of balance and harmony. This approach moves beyond the traditional biomedical model of disease management, embracing the science of energy, intention, and love as fundamental healing forces.

Drawing from quantum physics, neuroplasticity, epigenetics, and consciousness research, this theory asserts that thoughts, emotions, and intentions are powerful forces capable of shaping reality. Just as quantum computing transcends binary logic, allowing for infinite possibilities, so too does the human mind operate beyond conventional limits—holding the potential to influence healing at the deepest levels.

In this paradigm, intention, prayer, meditation, and visualization are not abstract concepts but scientifically supported practices that activate the body's innate ability to heal. Nurses, as facilitators of healing, can use these techniques to create environments that nurture the physical, emotional, and spiritual well-being of their patients. By integrating complementary therapies such as acupuncture, energy healing, sound therapy, and breathwork, nursing shifts from a mechanistic approach to one that harnesses the power of life force energy for optimal health.

The Universal Connectivity Theory, rooted in both quantum science and spiritual wisdom, proposes that everything in existence is interwoven through an intelligent field of energy. This field, often described as Universal Intelligence or Divine Consciousness, governs the symmetry of the cosmos, the harmony of nature, and the profound interconnectedness of all life.

Love, as the highest vibrational frequency, is the force that binds this universal fabric together. Across cultures and faith traditions, love is described not just as an emotion but as the essence of creation itself—the force through which healing, transformation, and unity occur. In nursing, this means shifting from a purely clinical perspective to one that acknowledges the profound impact of human connection, compassion, and intention in healing.

Research in heart-brain coherence, quantum entanglement, and neurobiology supports the idea that states of love, gratitude, and mindfulness alter physiological responses, reduce stress, and enhance the body's natural healing mechanisms. Dr. Joe Dispenza's work in neuroplasticity, for example, has demonstrated how aligning thoughts and emotions with elevated states of love and coherence can activate self-healing mechanisms at the genetic level.

Similarly, the Wim Hof Method has proven that individuals can consciously influence their autonomic nervous system, demonstrating the power of breath, mindset, and cold therapy in enhancing immunity, reducing inflammation, and improving overall health. These findings reinforce the New Nursing Theory's assertion that nurses must go beyond treating symptoms and instead guide patients toward holistic healing through intentional energy work.

Quantum mechanics has shown us that small shifts in initial conditions can create large, unpredictable transformations—a concept echoed in the Butterfly Effect. In healthcare, this principle suggests that every interaction, thought, and intention of a nurse can ripple through the patient's energy field, influencing their recovery trajectory.

Quantum Entanglement & Healing – Just as two entangled particles influence each other across vast distances, nurses and patients share an energetic bond, where intentional care and love can facilitate healing beyond physical touch. Superposition & Possibility – Patients exist in a state of infinite potential—by holding the highest intention for healing, nurses can influence the outcome in powerful, yet subtle ways. Resonance & Coherence – Love and compassion create harmonic resonance in the body's energy system, aligning all aspects of the self—physical, mental, emotional, and spiritual—toward a state of well-being.

By recognizing the interplay between consciousness, energy, and healing, nurses can intentionally participate in shaping patient outcomes. Through mindfulness, collaborative care, visualization, and sound therapy, they create high-frequency healing environments that amplify the body's ability to regenerate and thrive.

The New Nursing Theory challenges us to redefine healing, not as a mechanical process, but as a co-creative act between patient, nurse, and the Universal Field of Love. Whether through quantum physics, ancient healing traditions, or modern neuroscience, the evidence is clear: the mind shapes health, and love is the ultimate healer.

As healthcare evolves, the integration of energy medicine, lifestyle interventions, and consciousness-based healing will become essential in managing chronic diseases and reducing healthcare costs. By teaching patients to harness the power of mindfulness, visualization, and positive affirmations, nurses empower them to take control of their health and align with the limitless intelligence of the universe.

Ultimately, everything in the universe is energy, and as nurses, we have the profound responsibility of ensuring that this energy is directed toward healing, harmony, and love. In doing so, we not only transform individual lives but elevate the entire profession of nursing into a higher state of consciousness and care.

---

[i] http://samples.jbpub.com/9781284091502/Sitzman3e_CH03_Sample.pdf

[ii] https://www.watsoncaringscience.org/jean-bio/caring-science-theory/#10cp

*Watson's Caring Science & Human Caring Theory*

[iii] Hofstadter, Douglas R., and Emmanuel Sander. *Surfaces and Essences: Analogy as the Fuel and Fire of Thinking.* New York: Basic Books, 2013, p. 135. See also Pinker, Steven. *The Stuff of Thought: Language as a Window into Human Nature.* New York: Viking, 2007.

[iv] Kristin Barton Cuthriell, MEd, MSW, LCSW. Intentional Thinking. The Snowball Effect. 2016: https://thesnowballeffect.com/2016/05/18/intentional-thinking/

[v] *Greg Kestin, How Much Does a Thought Weigh? 2017 PBS Nova video:* https://www.pbs.org/wgbh/nova/video/how-much-does-a-thought-weigh/

[vi] *Neville Goddard. Is Your Mind Sending Signals Without You Knowing? The Law of Thought Transmission:* https://tammy.ai/keypoints/self-improvement/mindfulness-and-meditation/unlocking-the-power-of-thought-3

[vii] https://www.webmd.com/mental-health/positive-thinking-overview

[viii] Byrne (2010) explores the power of love in her book "The Power", and discusses how it can be used to bring about desired outcomes.

[ix] Jean Watson: Theory of Human Caring. Angelo Gonzalo, BSN, RN. 2024: https://nurseslabs.com/jean-watsons-philosophy-theory-transpersonal-caring/

[x] https://www.linkedin.com/pulse/power-positive-thinking-sa-mi-iq86e/

[xi] https://www.linkedin.com/pulse/5-scientific-studies-prove-power-positive-thinking-mark-guidi/

[xii] https://www.mentalhelp.net/blogs/the-science-of-affirmations/

[xiii] https://www.ncbi.nlm.nih.gov/pmc/articles/PMC7166246/

[xiv] Farnam Street. (2019, November 27). *The butterfly effect: Everything you need to know about this powerful mental model.* https://fs.blog/2017/08/the-butterfly-effect/

[xv] Lena Wiklund Gustin RN, PhD, Lynne Wagner EdD, RN, MSN: *The butterfly effect of caring – clinical nursing teachers' understanding of self-compassion as a source to compassionate care*, (2012), The Authors Scandinavian Journal of Caring Sciences 2012 Nordic College of Caring Science.

Halpern, P. (2018, February 14). *Chaos theory, the butterfly effect, and the computer glitch that started it all.*

Forbes. https://www.forbes.com/sites/startswithabang/2018/02/13/chaos-theory-the-butterfly-effect-and-the-computer-glitch-that-started-it-all/#1c89e3f269f6

Davey, B. (2011, October 6). *Economics is not a social science.* Resilience. https://www.resilience.org/stories/2011-10-07/economics-not-social-science/

Flam, F. (2012, June 15). *The Physics of Ray Bradbury's "A Sound of Thunder".* The Philadelphia Inquierer. https://www.inquirer.com/philly/blogs/evolution/Time-and-The-Physics-of-Ray-Bradbury

[xvi] National Alliance on Mental Illness. Critical things to know about emotions for mental health and healing.

[xvii] An S, Ji LJ, Marks M, Zhang Z. Two sides of emotion: Exploring positivity and negativity in six basic emotions across cultures. Front Psychol. 2017;8:610. doi:10.3389/fpsyg.2017.00610

[xviii] Arslanoglou E, Banerjee S, Pantelides J, Evans L, Kiosses DN. Negative emotions and the course of depression during psychotherapy in suicidal older adults with depression and cognitive impairment. *The American Journal of Geriatric Psychiatry.* 2019;27(12):1287-1295. doi:10.1016/j.jagp.2019.08.018

[xix] Lamers SM, Bolier L, Westerhof GJ, Smit F, Bohlmeijer ET. The impact of emotional well-being on long-term recovery and survival in physical illness: a meta-analysis. *J Behav Med.* 2012;35(5):538-547. doi:10.1007/s10865-011-9379-8

[xx] National Institutes of Health. Lingering feelings over daily stresses may impact long-term health.

[xxi] Boguszewski, K., & Zalewska, M. (2020). Mindfulness and self-care in chronic illness. Journal of Health Psychology, 25(5), 673-684. doi: 10.1177/1359105318755261

[xxii] Prabhakar, H., & Damodaran, A. (2021). Mindfulness and self-compassion: Exploring pathways to adolescent resilience. Children and Youth Services Review, 125, 106028. doi: 10.1016/j.childyouth.2021.106028

[xxiii] Talaee, N., & Najafi, G. (2018). The effects of positive thinking on self-care behaviors in patients with type 2 diabetes: A randomized controlled trial. Diabetes & Metabolic Syndrome: Clinical Research & Reviews, 12(1), 75-80. doi: 10.1016/j.dsx.2017.08.011

[xxiv] Lengacher, C. A., Reich, R. R., Post-White, J., Moscoso, M. S., Shelton, M. M., Barta, M. K., ... & Goodman, M. (2018). Mindfulness based stress reduction (MBSR (BC)) in breast cancer survivors: symptom outcomes and biomarkers. Cancer Nursing, 41(4), 271-278.

[xxv] Janssen M, Heerkens Y, Kuijer W, van der Heijden B, Engels J. Effects of Mindfulness-Based Stress Reduction on employees' mental health: A systematic review. PLoS One. 2018 Jan 24;13(1):e0191332. doi: 10.1371/journal.pone.0191332. PMID: 29364935; PMCID: PMC5783379.

[xxvi] Matos LC, Machado JP, Monteiro FJ, Greten HJ. Understanding Traditional Chinese Medicine Therapeutics: An Overview of the Basics and Clinical Applications. Healthcare (Basel). 2021 Mar 1;9(3):257. doi: 10.3390/healthcare9030257. PMID: 33804485; PMCID: PMC8000828.

www.ingramcontent.com/pod-product-compliance
Lightning Source LLC
Chambersburg PA
CBHW071235070526
44583CB00017B/2188